CW00741648

THE
PMT
SOLUTION

THE PMT SOLUTION

Premenstrual Tension:

The Nutritional Approach

by Dr. Ann Nazzaro
& Dr. Donald Lombard
with Dr. David Horrobin

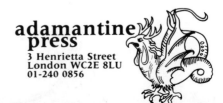

adamantine
press
3 Henrietta Street
London WC2E 8LU
01-240 0856

ISBN 0–7449–0001–8

Copyright © 1985 Eden Press. Published by arrangment. All rights reserved. No part of this book may be reproduced, stored in a retrieval system, or transmitted in any form or by any means, electronic, mechanical, photocopying, recording or otherwise, without the written permission of the publisher.

The information in this book is meant to complement the advice and guidance of your physician; it is not a substitute for a professional opinion. Because this book discusses a wide variety of situations, you should keep in mind that the information presented may not apply to your particular case. Before following any suggestions or course of treatment, you should consult your physician.

Credits: Cover design: Luba Zagurak with D. O'Leary; Cover photo: David Laforge; Cover model: Nancy Hood; Book design: D. O'Leary with Evelyne Hertel

First published in 1985
In Great Britain by
Adamantine Press, 3 Henrietta Street, London WC2E 8LU
In Canada by
Eden Press, 4626 St. Catherine St. W., Montreal H3Z 1S3
In the United States by
Winston Press, 430 Oak Grove, Minneapolis, MN 55403

British Library Cataloguing in Publication

Nazzaro, Anne
   The PMT solution: premenstrual tension: the nutritional
   approach
1. Premenstrual Syndrome
I. Title. II. Lombard, Donald. III. Horrobin, David.
618.1'72   RG165

ISBN 0–7449–001–8

A NOTE FROM THE AUTHORS

We will refer to PMT, Premenstrual Tension, as PMS, Premenstrual Syndrome, throughout this book. We prefer the term PMS because it better represents the entire spectrum of symptoms that may be experienced by PMT sufferers.

Not all of the products mentioned in this book are available in all countries.

DEDICATION

The history of medicine is replete with instances of emotional illness thought to have psychological causes and subsequently discovered to have organic or well-defined physical causes. Chronic metal poisons and thyroid illnesses are classic examples of these tragic errors.

We, the authors of this book, believe that yet another psychological illness has given way to medical progress and found to be the result of a well-defined physical abnormality occurring within the metabolism of the brain and body. That illness is commonly referred to as *Pre-Menstrual Syndrome* (PMS) or *Pre-Menstrual Tension* (PMT). Untold hours, days and portions of every month have been a physical and emotional disaster for thousands of women because of PMS.

This book is an attempt to tell the story of some recent research that has demonstrated the physical abnormality and metabolism imbalance causing the difficulty, and to show what can be done to help the majority of women who have this illness.

With many colleagues in the field of psychiatry, we share the discomfort of having called many women "psychiatric" when they were not. We didn't believe them—even when they often insisted that they were telling the truth.

It is to these women—from whom we ask more patience than we gave—that we humbly dedicate this book.

ACKNOWLEDGEMENTS

We would like to thank the following people for their assistance, support and encouragement in making this book a reality: Sherri Clarkson, Pamela Chichinskas, Fawn Duchaine, Evelyne Hertel, Cynthia Taupier, Anne Lombard, Pamela Lombard, Karen Lombard, John Moriarty, Laurianne Fiorentino, and Amy Zeldes.

Our grateful thanks to Cathy Lebow Axelson, assistant editor for New England's *Advocate* newspapers, without whose invaluable help this book would never have been written.

TABLE OF CONTENTS

FOREWORD

Ann Nazzaro (Ph.D., United States International University) and Donald R. Lombard (M.D., Boston University School of Medicine) first worked together in 1975 as staff members at Baystate Medical Center in Springfield, Massachusetts. Lombard was Director of Psychiatric Outpatient Services, and Nazzaro was outpatient-therapist and Emergency Services Crisis clinician. A year or so later, while Nazzaro was in California working on her Ph.D. in clinical psychology, Dr. Lombard became especially interested in the biochemistry of depression and implemented a psychopharmacology program at Baystate that focused on the treatment of depression. He then convinced Nazzaro to return to New England to collaborate on clinical research in the psychobiology of depression.

Lombard noticed that a number of successful depression treatment programs based on the use of psychotropic medications were subject to relapse. Through a friend and colleague, Julien Lieb, M.D. (then at Yale University), he came upon a series of references on the work of David Horrobin, Ph.D., M.D., a medical researcher in Montreal specializing in the metabolism of nutrition and related chronic health problems. Through Lieb, Lombard and Nazzaro were introduced to Horrobin. They were impressed by Horrobin's findings, and, based on his research, began using a nutritional approach to depression.

i

They found the effects of prostaglandin-regulating nutrients for the treatment of depression in women and men to be impressive—often reversing relapses. The most startling discovery, however, was that women who took prostaglandin-regulating nutrients began to experience a marked diminution of premenstrual tension. The women started to describe how calm and at ease they felt, and how different this was for them. Before taking the nutrients, the women explained, they could always predict when their periods would begin based solely on their physical and emotional state. Now, they told Lombard and Nazzaro, they were finding themselves pleasantly surprised as they were no longer able to predict when they would menstruate because there was no longer any warning.

Then Nazzaro, who was also premenstrual and had problems every month with bloating and mood swings, tried the nutritional program on herself. It worked. Nazzaro's experiences with treating her own premenstrual syndrome formed the basis of the program subsequently developed for PMS by means of prostaglandin-regulation through nutrients.

A fascinating footnote to the story related to Horrobin's research. Horrobin had unintentionally come upon the interrelation of the prostaglandins and premenstrual syndrome. At that time, he was looking into the effects of prolactin, a pituitary hormone that regulates the production of progesterone and stimulates the mammary glands. During the course of his research Horrobin injected himself with prolactin on several different occasions. He swelled up, felt irritable and "fed up with it all." His experiences, he says today, were remarkably like those of women having premenstrual syndrome. He suggests, only half humorously, that he may be the only male in history to have been "premenstrual."

In his laboratory work, Horrobin found that essential fatty acids are an intrinsic part of premenstrual syndrome regulation; and that vitamin B6 is necessary as a co-factor for the conversion to take place.

Further research revealed the role of gammalinolenic acid (GLA), an essential fatty acid that appears during the process of conversion (but which must be ingested separately in some cases). Despite extensive research, GLA has been found present in sufficient quantitites to be used effectively in only two sources at present: human breast milk and the seed oil of the evening primrose plant. Horrobin also found that co-factors other than vitamin B6 play an essential role in the conversion process.

Based on Horrobin's theoretical and laboratory work, and on the initial clinical success of Lombard and Nazzaro, independent clinical trials were initiated in the late '70s and early '80s. Early results were very favorable. Since then, Horrobin has continued research on the use of prostaglandin-regulating nutrients for other health problems, and Lombard and Nazzaro have developed and refined the nutritional solution to PMS. They have also expanded their use of prostaglandin-regulating nutrients and vitamin and mineral supplements to the treatment of various problems once thought to be psychological, or even psychosomatic in origin, such as hyperactivity in children. Their other field of concentration is the treatment of immune system dysfunction, specifically enviromental and food allergies.

This book has been designed to augment and/or facilitate direct care by health professionals. The authors cannot take any medical or legal responsibility. You, your physician, or the health professional who examines and treats you must take the responsibility for the use made of this information.

THE
PMT
SOLUTION

THE BIOCHEMISTRY OF PMS

by David F. Horrobin
Efamol Research Institute,
Kentville, Nova Scotia, Canada

Premenstrual syndrome (PMS) is a condition that has become widely recognized by the medical profession only during the past ten years, largely through the efforts of one woman, a British doctor, Katharina Dalton. PMS was described many years earlier, but obstetricians, gynecologists and family practitioners ignored what had been written about it.

Part of the problem is that MDs are trained to identify illnesses by looking at the symptoms that occur. One group of symptoms means one illness, another group of symptoms means another illness. But the range of symptoms found in PMS was so broad, and the differences between women so great that many doctors had difficulty believing that a real illness was involved. The symptoms fell into three broad categories.

PHYSICAL SYMPTOMS

Weight gain, abdominal bloating, ankle swelling, breast swelling, breast pain and tenderness, a feeling of pelvic fullness, dragging pain, thirst, and reduced urine production were all described, even though there were often striking differences from woman to woman.

PSYCHO-LOGICAL SYMPTOMS

Anxiety, tension, depression, weepiness, anger and paranoia were also described, but again, the precise symptoms varied from woman to woman.

OTHER SYMPTOMS

An astonishing variety of other symptoms have been described. They include loss of sex drive (or more rarely, an excessive sex drive), food cravings, headache, clumsiness, worsening of skin problems in those with a tendency to bad skin, asthmatic attacks in those with asthma, and even epileptic attacks in those known to have epilepsy.

Almost any symptom may occur in PMS. The key to diagnosis is the recognition that symptoms always occur before menstruation and are always relieved by menstruation. The following are the common ones:

Table 1: Symptoms of PMS

- Anxiety, tension, worry
- Irritability, hostility, anger
- Depression, tiredness, unhappiness, crying
- Food cravings
- Swelling of the abdomen
- Swollen ankles
- Swollen, tender and painful breasts
- Weight gain
- Headache
- Skin breaking out
- Painful joints or back

To some extent, one can sympathize with the doctors. Faced with such an astonishing variety of symptoms without any common theme or apparent common basis, the temptation to dismiss the whole thing as a lot of nonsense is very strong. It was Dr. Dalton's particular contribution to note and to stress that there was a single unifying feature of PMS that allowed it to be identified. This was the *timing* of the symptoms. PMS is a condition that is identified not by *which* symptoms occur, but by *when* they occur. PMS is defined by the occurrence of symptoms that develop or worsen substantially in the two weeks before menstruation is expected and that disappear or improve dramatically in the 48 hours (and often within the one or two hours) after menstrual-blood flow has started. It is *the relief by menstruation* that is the key factor and what distinguishes PMS from the other common menstrual cycle disorder, dysmenorrhea (period pains). Dysmenorrhea begins as or just *before* menstrual flow begins. PMS ends as or just *after* menstrual flow begins. The two must be clearly distinguished because they respond to quite different treatments.

So, almost any symptom can be an aspect of PMS if the timing is right. By far the most common symptoms are those in the first two groups, but individual women may well experience any of the others.

THEORIES OF PMS

The theories of PMS can be roughly divided into three groups. First, there is the view that PMS does not exist and that it is a non-illness. This was the view held by most doctors until rather recently. Women with PMS were thought to be neurotic. It is my suspicion that the explosion of tranquillizer use in the 1960s and 1970s can, to a very substantial degree, be attributed to PMS. Women with PMS complained of a wide variety of psychological symptoms, were held to be neurotic, and were given pills to calm them down. As a result, they ended up being tranquillized all month for an illness that caused problems for only one or two weeks per month, and their physical symptoms were unchanged. This type of treatment leads to women denying symptoms that are undoubtedly real, and attempting to cope with a problem that can be dealt with very successfully, as Drs. Lombard and Nazzaro demonstrate in this book. It is about as sensible as telling women that menstruation does not exist and can be ignored without taking precautions to do something about the flow of blood.

Second, there is a view that PMS does exist but is purely a psychological problem related to fear of menstruation. This theory suggests that menstruation in our society is surrounded by so many irrational ideas and superstitions that some women become terrified of it. As the time of each menstrual period approaches, they therefore become more and more distressed in anticipation of the problems it might bring.

This theory has three major problems that its proponents have never seriously answered. First, if PMS is fear of menstruation, why are so many women delighted when menstruation comes, relieving all their PMS symptoms within a matter of hours? Second, what is the mechanism whereby such a psychological symptom can so often produce a range of unequivocal physical symptoms? A third problem for this theory is that PMS is actually relatively unusual among teenagers in the years after menstruation has just begun (when dysmenorrhea is very common). As the years go by, and especially with the birth of children, dysmenorrhea gets better and PMS gets worse. Perhaps the type of woman who is most severely affected by PMS is a woman in her 30s or early 40s with two or three children. This does not accord at all with the psychological explanations.

Third, there is the view that PMS is basically a disorder of body chemistry that leads to both physical and psychological problems. This is the position now held by almost everyone who has studied PMS seriously and who has had any experience of actually treating women with PMS. As yet, however, there is little agreement as to what actually is wrong.

Table 2: Theories of PMS

1. It doesn't exist.
2. Fear of menstruation
3. Biochemical theories: –progesterone deficiency;
    –low progesterone/ estrogen ratio;
    –high prolactin level;
    –abnormal endorphin production;
    –essential fatty acid problem.

Physical Theories

PMS occurs in what is known as the *luteal* phase of the menstrual cycle — when the ovaries are most active in producing female hormones. These hormones are of two main types, the estrogens, which are responsible for many of the female characteristics—including such things as body shape, skin quality, and maintenance of the reproductive tract; and progesterone, which joins forces with the estrogens to prepare the female body for the beginning of pregnancy and which plays a vital role in maintaining pregnancy through to the end.

Table 3: Actions of Estrogens and Progesterone
Estrogen

- Normal development at puberty of breasts, uterus and other reproductive organs.
- Normal female behavior.
- Normal building-up of the uterus in the first half of the menstrual cycle ready for ovulation.

Progesterone

- Building up uterus with estrogen in second half of menstrual cycle ready for pregnancy.
- Pregnancy hormone, making body ready for pregnancy with breast development, weight changes, water balance changes.
- Mild sedation.

Since these two types of hormones are produced in large amounts just when PMS occurs, it is natural to think that they are in some way the cause of PMS. This idea is reinforced by the fact that PMS usually does not disappear when the uterus is removed at hysterectomy so long as the ovaries remain intact. Even though there can be no actual menstruation after a hysterectomy, the cyclical physical symptoms and mood changes continue as before. If the ovaries are removed, however, PMS usually disappears with the cyclical hormonal changes that the ovaries bring about whether or not the uterus is present.

But there is an obvious problem in saying that the cyclical hormone changes *cause* PMS. This is that these cyclical hormonal changes occur in all menstruating women, whereas obviously symptomatic PMS occurs in less than half, and severe PMS only in about one woman in ten. So the hormone changes themselves cannot cause PMS because if they did, all menstruating women would have PMS.

Since the hormones must be involved in some way, Dr. Dalton proposed the theory that the real culprit was an abnormality in the ratio between the estrogens and progesterone. In particular, a deficiency of progesterone coupled with normal or elevated estrogen levels, and thus a low progesterone/estrogen ratio, was proposed as the cause of PMS. This is an attractive theory, but unfortunately, there is no evidence that it is true. Certainly there are some reports of low progesterone and/or high estrogen levels in some patients with PMS. Equally, however, there are some reports of exactly the opposite, and even more reports of a failure to find any difference in hormones between women with and without PMS. The consensus, therefore, is that there is no abnormality of these two hormones that can explain PMS. This view is reinforced by the failure of progesterone therapy (see later sections).

There are other hormones whose levels change during the menstrual cycle. They include prolactin, the hormone that is involved in controlling the breasts, and the morphine-like endorphins, which regulate mood among other things. I first became interested in prolactin and PMS when I injected myself with prolactin and became depressed, bloated, thirsty, and had reduced urine flow. However, while some women with PMS do have elevated prolactin levels and do improve when given bromocriptine (a drug that suppresses prolactin secretion), in most women with PMS, prolactin levels are in the normal range. Similarly, there is as yet no real evidence that women with PMS have any abnormality of endorphin levels.

In summary, the hormone changes that occur during the menstrual cycle are undoubtedly necessary if PMS is to develop. Yet there is no real evidence that the hormone levels in PMS are anything out of the ordinary. It therefore seems that there must be something else wrong in women with PMS that makes them unusually susceptible to the actions of perfectly normal menstrual cycle hormone changes. There is increasing evidence that that something is a minor abnormality in the way in which the body handles a group of essential nutrients known as the *essential fatty acids*, or EFAs.

EFAs and PMS

The main EFA in the diet is a substance called *linoleic acid* (LA). LA is in fact a type of vitamin, because it must be provided in food and cannot be made by the body. In a sense it is a pre-vitamin, because once in the body it is converted to a whole range of other important substances, including the ones shown below.

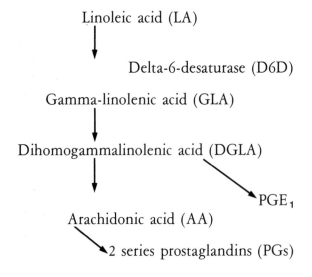

Linoleic acid (LA)

Delta-6-desaturase (D6D)

Gamma-linolenic acid (GLA)

Dihomogammalinolenic acid (DGLA)

PGE$_1$

Arachidonic acid (AA)

2 series prostaglandins (PGs)

Table 4: Functions of Essential Fatty Acids

- Necessary for the normal structure of all cell membranes throughout the body.
- Building blocks from which prostaglandins are made.
- Required for: smooth and supple, non-greasy skin; normal hair; normal brain function; normal heart and circulation; normal kidney function; normal function of ovaries and hormones; normal breast development and function; normal control of pain and inflammation.

LA, GLA, and AA are all known as EFAs. They seem to play vital roles in the structure of the body, since they are key components of every tissue and essential parts of the membranes around and within all the cells of the body. The prostaglandins (PGs), on the other hand, which are made from the EFAs, are short-lived regulating substances that control the behavior of all the body's organs.

It is therefore obvious that the chemical processes by which the body handles dietary LA are vital. Particularly important is the first step, the conversion of LA to GLA, which is carried out by an enzyme (a biochemical processing device) known as delta-6-desaturase (D6D). If anything is wrong with the D6D, then the body may be unable to use dietary LA normally.

In the context of PMS, there appear to be two groups of factors that can influence D6D activity. One is genetic, which seems to result in some people having D6D that is less active than usual. The other group is environmental, a range of factors that can reduce the activity of even a fully normal enzyme, but that are likely to have a much greater effect in those who are unfortunate enough to have an enzyme that is underactive for genetic reasons.

Table 5
Factors influencing the enzyme D6D,
which converts linoleic acid to gamma linoleic acid.

- Linoleic: inhibited by genetic background of atopy;
- genetic background of PMS;
- stress hormones;
- sugar-rich diets;
- lack of zinc, magnesium, or pyridoxine.

Atopy is a technical term doctors use to indicate a condition in which there is an increased risk of developing conditions such as eczema, asthma, hay fever and allergic rhinitis. The way in which atopy is inherited is not at all clear, but there is no doubt at all that it runs in families. It must be stressed that what is inherited is not eczema, or asthma, but simply an increased susceptibility to these conditions. In order for the illness to develop, the susceptible person must interact with something in the environment. It is this interaction that produces the actual illness. Some people may have the inherited atopic susceptibility, but are fortunate enough not to develop the actual illness because they have never encountered the environmental conditions that will make it emerge.

It is the impression of many doctors who see women with PMS that they have an unusually high frequency of eczema, asthma and allergies—either in themselves or in their immediate families. This was studied formally by a group of researchers in France; they found that the majority of women with severe PMS were atopic.

This is important because it is now known that atopic individuals have a minor problem with the D6D enzyme. In their blood, levels of linoleic acid are normal or often slightly above normal, indicating that there is nothing wrong with their nutritional intake of LA. In spite of that, levels of GLA, DGLA and AA are well below normal, suggesting that there is a problem in converting LA to GLA. Giving GLA in the form of evening primrose oil led to improvements in eczema and also to a rise in the levels of GLA, DGLA and AA.

Measurements of these fatty acids in women with PMS have now shown exactly the same problem as in the people with atopic eczema. This is not surprising, since the French study showed such a close association between atopy and PMS. Blood samples from women with PMS in London, England; Cardiff, Wales; Dundee, Scotland; and Lund, Sweden, have all been shown to have normal LA, yet low GLA, DGLA and AA.

Studies have also shown that these fatty acid abnormalities are present all the time, not just when the PMS symptoms are present. So these abnormalities, just like the normal changes in hormone levels, cannot be the *cause* of PMS by themselves. What seems to be the problem is that the abnormal fatty acid levels make a woman exceptionally sensitive to perfectly normal hormonal changes. Hormones that have no adverse effects in a woman with normal fatty acid levels can produce the full range of PMS symptoms in a woman whose fatty acid concentrations are abnormal. It is the *interaction* between the two that matters. Of course, because many women with PMS are atopic, allergies and other manifestations of atopy are common and may exaggerate the effect of the PMS or produce symptoms quite apart from the PMS.

Among the environmental factors that can effect the D6D, five appear to be particularly important. These may have little adverse action in those with a fully normal D6D, but if they act on individuals with a minor, genetically based D6D problem, or if several of the factors act together, they could produce abnormal fatty acid biochemistry. These factors are:

Stress

Under stress one produces a hormone called epinephrine (adrenaline) from the adrenal gland. Epinephrine inhibits the D6D, thus decreasing conversion of LA to GLA.

Simple Sugars

Animals fed diets rich in refined sugar show reduced D6D activity and a reduced ability to convert LA to GLA. It is probable that the same thing happens in humans. Sugar in drinks or on foods, and in candies, cookies and many other processed foods may have this effect.

Processed Vegetable Oils

Processing vegetable oils, to make them solid so they can be used in hard margarines and in shortening, converts the natural fatty acids into unusual *trans* forms. These have weak effects in blocking the D6D, which probably do not matter if the D6D is fully active. If, however, the D6D is not fully active, the trans acids may cause serious problems.

Magnesium

This essential mineral is required for the D6D to work normally. Women with PMS have been shown to have low magnesium levels in their blood.

Vitamin B6 (Pyridoxine)

This vitamin seems to be important for the D6D, and even more so for the conversion of GLA to DGLA.

Thus the latest evidence suggests that women with PMS have low levels of GLA, DGLA, and AA, probably in part because of a minor genetic abnormality in the

D6D. Stress, diets rich in sugar, and magnesium deficiency have all been reported in PMS and may exaggerate any underlying problem. Everyone in North America eats around 0.2 to 0.5 ounces (5 to 15 grams) of trans acids per day. These may not matter much in normal people, but may have a harmful effect in those with reduced D6D activity. Pyridoxine deficiency has not been shown to be present in PMS, but there is no doubt that many women do better with daily supplements of pyridoxine. Such doses may be helping the body to make the most of what fatty acids are available.

The fatty acid problems thus appear to make a woman susceptible to perfectly normal hormonal changes so that it is the *interaction* that causes the problems.

Table 6: Proposed Mechanism of PMS

- Hormone levels are normal. There is nothing fundamentally wrong with the menstrual cycle or reproduction.
- There is a minor abnormality of EFA metabolism leading to a failure to make GLA from linoleic acid normally.
- Levels of GLA and other fatty acids are low. This leads to exceptional sensitivity to hormones, so that normal hormones produce abnormal effects.

TREATMENT Patients with almost any disease, including serious conditions such as cancer or arthritis, will get better, at least temporarily, if they *believe* they are going to get better. Hundreds of studies have shown that patients with serious diseases will improve if they are given a dummy (placebo) tablet, capsule, or injection. This may be difficult for lay people to believe, but it is something that every doctor knows about. This is why doctors are often so skeptical when they are told that a patient has gotten better after some new treatment.

The doctor knows that the patient might have improved even if the new treatment was completely useless.

This is why doctors insist on placebo-controlled studies before they can be convinced about the value of a new treatment. In a placebo-controlled study, half the patients are given active tablets, capsules or injections. The other half are given materials identical in appearance but containing totally inert substances. Neither the doctor nor the patients know who is getting what. The results of the treatment in each patient are carefully analyzed and only after that is the code broken so that the doctor knows who was on the real treatment and who on the dummy.

The first thing that astonishes people who do such trials is that almost always, the patients in the placebo group show substantial improvement. Improvement thus occurs when almost any treatment is given by a doctor, even if completely inert substances are used. The test of whether a substance is having a real effect is whether the improvement in the active group is greater than that in the placebo group. Only then can it genuinely be said that the treatment itself is effective.

Progesterone

When considered in this rigorous way, very few treatments have been found to be effective in PMS. The most popular treatment of all is progesterone. This cannot satisfactorily be taken by mouth, and so has to be given by injections or by suppositories, methods of administration that have even larger placebo effects than medicines taken orally. Progesterone has been very heavily promoted—largely on the grounds of the unproven hypothesis that there is a deficiency of progesterone in PMS. There is no doubt that many women feel better with their first few courses of progesterone injections or suppositories. Equally, there is no doubt that placebo-controlled trials have shown that *progesterone is no better than placebo*. In fact, if anything, the progesterone group did *worse* than the placebo group. People who criticize the trials have said that the doses were too small. In fact, the doses were more than large enough to correct any conceivable progesterone deficiency. Progesterone is itself a tranquillizer and an anaesthetic, and the truly astronomical doses used by some clinics probably do make some women feel calmer, but equally probably, they are little more than very expensive tranquillizers with a wide range of side effects.

In contrast, pyridoxine has been shown, in a placebo-controlled study, to be effective in PMS, but only at doses that are far higher than those normally required for its use as a vitamin, but not large enough to cause any toxic symptoms.

Evening Primrose Oil

GLA in the form of evening primrose oil has now been shown to be effective in three different types of trials.

At St. Thomas's Hospital in London, England, Dr. Michael Brush conducted a trial in which over a hundred and fifty women who had failed with other methods of treatment were tested. Because these women had been treated previously and had failed to respond, they were unlikely to be people who would respond to placebo. Yet, in spite of this, two-thirds obtained complete relief from evening primrose oil, and another quarter obtained substantial though not complete relief. Only about 10 percent of the women in this very difficult group of patients failed to respond.

Placebo-controlled trials have been carried out in ordinary PMS by Dr. Brush in London, by Professor Olavi Ylikorkala at the University of Helsinki in Finland, and by Professor Per-Anne Ockermann at the University of Lund in Sweden. Studies in women whose main complaint was premenstrual breast pain and tenderness were carried out by Dr. Paul Preece at the University of Dundee in Scotland, and by Dr. Robert Mansel at the University of Wales in Cardiff. In all of these studies, without exception, evening primrose oil was shown to be better than placebo at relieving PMS symptoms.

Evening primrose oil is now used extensively by gynecological and family practitioners, especially in Britain and Scandinavia, for the treatment of PMS. When adequate doses are used, the success rate is consistently 50 to 90 percent, and unlike the effects of placebo, the response continues indefinitely. Many women find they can reduce their dose of evening primrose oil as time goes on, and still obtain full relief from their symptoms.

Thus evening primrose oil is by far the most solidly researched and simplest approach to treating PMS. On a weight basis, the doses are only about one-quarter to one-half of the GLA taken in daily by a fully breast-fed baby. Moreover, evening primrose oil is able to restore to normal the abnormal EFA levels seen in PMS.

PMS is a real condition; it is not "all in the mind." In most women, however, it seems to be a relatively simple nutritional problem that does not require treatment with hormones or drugs. As outlined in this book, most women should be able to work with their doctors over a period of months to obtain complete control over their symptoms.

"WHO ARE YOU TODAY?"

Elizabeth F. was a terrific waitress, the best the restaurant ever had for two, maybe two-and-a-half weeks of the month. For the rest of the month, she was the worst. She became rude, irritable, and downright nasty to customers and co-workers.

"It was just awful," Elizabeth recalls. "I was so short-tempered, and I had these hot flashes. Then I'd break out in a cold sweat." She knew she was being unreasonable, but couldn't help it. "One minute everything would be fine, and then the next, I'd be crying." Elizabeth was depressed and forgetful. She also felt fat. Every month, she bloated up by as much as six pounds and, as a result, she had to have an extra set of clothes on hand. At this point, she was taking about six Tylenol pills daily.

While the restaurant could ill-afford to lose its best waitress, neither could it afford to keep someone with Jekyll-and-Hyde mood swings. "Who are you today?" the rest of the kitchen staff would jokingly ask when Elizabeth came in. She couldn't take her own irritability much longer either, and felt she was heading for a breakdown.

Regularly, her breasts became so sore that when her five-year-old tried to snuggle up for a hug, she recoiled in pain and pushed the child off her lap. The children were having a hard time trying to understand their mother, who sometimes played with them, read stories out loud and was sweet and loving, and who, at other times would turn on them angrily for no apparent reason. Elizabeth had recently remarried and was working hard at establishing a good relationship.

It was a crowded day at the restaurant when an elderly couple came in. They were seated at one of Elizabeth's tables, and it seemed as if no time at all had passed before they called her over demanding menus and water.

"Can't you wait a minute?" she raged. "What do I look like, Superwoman?"

"That did it," Elizabeth told us when she came in shortly after for a first consultation. "I need help." Elizabeth was diagnosed as having PMS.

A daily regimen of primrose oil, 50-balance vitamin B complex, zinc, and half an aspirin worked almost immediately to minimize her premenstrual moodiness. By her next pre-time, the results were already apparent. She remained, for the most part, her better self.

"My children, my husband and my boss all noticed . . . that I'm more in control of myself and that my temper isn't so bad," she said with pride. After her period was over she announced that "it was the best I've ever had." By that she meant that it was the most ordinary, least noticeable and most "nothing" period she had experienced.

Over the course of the next year, the nutrient program was altered slightly to provide her with an individually tailored, optimal combination of vitamins and dosages. Elizabeth not only feels better now; she even looks different. When she first came in, she had a tired, stressed look, with dark circles under the eyes and a heavy, weighted powerlessness to her. Her posture and movements gave the impression of someone on the verge of the dark abyss, a person about to throw in the towel. Now she sports a lovely smile and moves with natural energy. A gentleness shows at the corners of her eyes where strain and disappointment had shown before. She is one of our first success stories, a typical case of PMS successfully diagnosed and treated.

Esther L. saw us on a TV talk-show interview. Esther was an accountant working with a major pharmaceutical house—an extremely energetic and ambitious career woman. But for the last six months, she told us, she'd been suffering tremendously from migraine headaches that regularly descended upon her 10 to 14 days before the onset of her period. In addition, she was subject to mood swings, irritability, breast tenderness, bloating, reduced libido and constipation. Thirty-seven years old, Esther was another classic case of premenstrual syndrome.

"This," she stated "is definitely getting in the way of my career. Especially when I suddenly get a migraine during board meetings or conferences. I love the intensity of my work, but I can't have that kind of problem picking away at my performance. I never know when it will hit."

Esther had already tried several solutions for her complaints. Initially, biofeedback had helped, but then it seemed to lose its effectiveness. She was already taking vitamin B_6, chlorophyll tablets, vitamin B-complex, vitamin C, and bran. She ate a relatively clean, additive-free diet, and avoided processed foods, sugar, salt, and other foods associated with migraines.

Because her symptoms increased noticeably whenever she ate chocolate, we suspected that she had premenstrual syndrome aggravated by allergies. We started her on a program of vitamin B_6, zinc, vitamin C, vitamin B-complex, and evening primrose oil.

One month later, Esther was back at our offices. "My energy is 50 percent better, bloating is 50 percent better, breast tenderness 50 percent better," she reported efficiently. (Esther is always analytical and very direct.) "My constipation is about 70 percent improved. I'm handling stress better now, and my irritability has improved dramatically. I seem to require one hour less sleep at night. And I didn't have a headache at all last month. In general," she summed up, "I feel much better."

Eventually, we found Esther's food allergies included not only chocolate, but rice and dairy foods as well. We treated her for all of them. Recently she sent us a newspaper clipping announcing her latest coup as head of the accounting department for a prestigious ad agency. "Thought you'd like to share my exciting news," she wrote. "I never could have done it without the sense of mental and physical well-being you've helped me reach."

INTRODUCTION

When someone has a variety of symptoms that do not seem related, symptoms that grow and change over a period of time, symptoms that are hard to pin down, he or she is highly likely to encounter confusion and hesitancy from the medical professional. Why? Because the problems these symptoms represent are still on the frontier of research. We are just beginning to learn about, to recognize and to treat what we call *system* or *whole system* diseases.

PMS is one of a variety of system diseases that usually "fall between the [medical] cracks." People will go from competent doctor to competent doctor without getting relief from these problems that have no name, are not widely understood, or are new in the lexicon of diseases. Allergies, *Candida* overgrowth, and PMS are all in this category. There are probably dozens of others we have not yet diagnosed or discovered the origins of.

Before illness is even recognized, the human body is going through a series of imbalances that should be termed *illness*. By the time symptoms become discernable, the body systems are well into the process of breakdown. The nebulous, hard-to-diagnose symptoms that come and go indicate that a breakdown is already underway. The downward spiral from relatively good health to disease has begun.

Our approach is to stop that fall, to prevent that breakdown before it can interfere with living—as it does in arthritis, allergies, PMS, and other system problems—and with the health of the individual. We are at the beginning of a major health revolution of which PMS and its treatment is one small part. For want of a better term, we refer to this changing medical approach as *nutritional pharmacology*.

This approach—the use of dietary (nutritional) means to correct imbalances in the biochemistry of the body—is an attempt to circumvent an underlying problem that seems to be endemic to our industrialized world: inadequate nutrition. This approach prescribes nutrients that are needed in greater supply due to increased need, often because they have been processed out of our foods, or because other chemicals in our environment are depleting them.

When the chemicals and nutrients that are missing are determined and then replaced, the changes are as dramatic as with any other "medicine," such as antibiotic or psychotropic drugs. Most people think of vitamins and nutrients as subtle, mysterious, and slow-working items. Sometimes they are, but they can be powerful and dramatic in their eventual effects.

To better understand our present state of nutrition, let's look at what our ancestors ate, how they ate it and when they ate it. Our primate ancestors probably go back at least seven million years, and we know that there were no substantial changes in their diet until at best twenty thousand years ago. More likely there were no real changes until five or ten thousand years ago. We have gone from the diet of primitive man to our present diet in a phenomenally short period of time. From over five thousand years ago until a few hundred years ago, dietary changes evolved over many generations, but in the last one hundred years—and especially in the last fifty—our diet has changed radically.

What have we done to our diet? In the last century alone, we have gone from an average consumption of 5 pounds (2.25 kg) of sugar a year to an average of 150 pounds (67.5 kg) a year. All of it is refined sugar. That's just one of a hundred changes. For instance, there are thousands of chemicals that end up in our food. Some of it is added on purpose, such as preservatives, coloring, flavorings, and other processing chemicals. Some of it is added indirectly, such as antibiotics that were fed to the animals we get our meat from, or pesticides that coat and penetrate our fruits, vegetables and grains.

It could be said that given the adaptability of humans, and with evolution as creative as it is, we would adapt to these chemicals if we had a hundred thousand years for the process. But we have been trying to adjust in only 50 years, and our bodies, our metabolism, just can't keep up.

One hundred years ago, there may not have been a chronic health problem such as PMS, or it may have affected only a very small percentage of the female population. Now, however, as we become inundated with toxic substances, our bodies are experiencing such increased biochemical stress that we are seeing an epidemic of problems. Hyperactivity in children, diabetes, arthritis, and cardiovascular diseases are among these problems and all are what we call the *lifestyle* diseases. All are indicative of the distress our bodies are experiencing.

It is our contention that good health today is more and more frequently a partnership between concerned professionals and educated consumers. It seems that in some areas at least, the cult of the expert—that paragon whose every word is unhesitatingly believed to be truth, until the paragon errs, even slightly—gives way, as Mark Gershon expressed it in *A Choice of Heroes*, to the ideal of the person who shares knowledge, the teacher who helps empower others. It is the shared responsibility today, of both physician and consumer, to learn, to teach, and to remain open to the evolution of knowledge.

1

WHAT IS PMS?

Premenstrual syndrome (PMS) is the cluster of symptoms that appear 2 to 14 days before the onset of a menstrual period. The symptoms are both physical and psychological, and they vary from person to person; they remain the same for any single individual over a number of cycles. One person may have only one or two symptoms, or several of them; her symptoms may also change over time.

"She's like a different person."

"I don't know what gets into me sometimes. It seems that everything I do is wrong. Nothing works out right."

"Something happens and I don't feel like myself. I get angry at small things that wouldn't normally bother me at all."

"I'm really terrible. I don't know how my family can stand me. I don't mean to be that way, and I always apologize after."

These are the kinds of statements one hears frequently from premenstrual women or their families or friends. Women with PMS don't require a calendar, neatly marked off, to tell them when they are going to get their period. When they begin to feel that the world is a terrible place to be, when "everything just seems to fall apart," when they feel depressed, lethargic, bloated, crampy and ugly, they know they'll menstruate in a few days, or a week, or however many days their pre-time usually lasts. They may not realize that this syndrome is anything out of the ordinary at all; they may not know that it is a recognized medical problem. But they do know that they feel bad.

Moreover, things seem to go wrong during the premenstrual time. It is also when 46 percent of women's psychiatric hospital admissions occur, and when 67 percent of women who are alcoholics begin a drinking binge. (To complicate this, alcohol has a more direct, powerful effect physiologically on women when they are premenstrual.) Fifty-two percent of women's hospital admissions from accidents (including car accidents) occur shortly before the onset of their menses. Forty-nine percent of female prisoners committed their crimes during PMS time. The greatest number of female suicide attempts are made during that part of their cycle. School girls get the worst grades and have the worst disciplinary problems during pre-times. School teachers who are premenstrual are stricter and more likely to punish the students than they are during the rest of the month.

The most common symptoms of PMS are:

Physical
- bloating
- breast tenderness/soreness
- lower back pain
- nausea, vomiting
- acne
- headaches, cramps
- lethargy, loss of energy

- fatigue, increased need for sleep, or insomnia, restlessness
- increased hunger, food cravings—especially for sweets, chocolates, or carbohydrates
- weight fluctuations

Psychological/Emotional

- depression
- crying spells
- anxiety
- mood swings, irritability
- increased or decreased sex drive
- decreased coping mechanisms
- uncontrollable outbursts of anger/hostility
- suicidal impulses
- lack of concentration
- memory lapses, confusion
- feelings of insecurity
- decreased feeling of self-worth

Other conditions typically associated with PMS, or aggravated at premenstrual time, include: dizziness, faintness, difficulty standing for long periods of time, migraine headaches, visual blind spots, aching varicose veins, chest pains, asthma attacks, constipation *or* diarrhea, colds and a runny nose, sinusitis, sore throat, hoarseness, loss of smell, thirst, arthritis and other joint problems, rheumatism, hypoglycemia, itchiness, greasy *or* dry hair, conjunctivitis and styes, problems with contact lenses, vaginal discharge, hemorrhoids, frequent need to urinate, epilepic seizures, herpes outbreaks, ringing in the ears, and alcoholic binges exacerbating chronic diseases such as ulcer, ulcerative colitis, and depression.

When a sample of premenstrual sufferers was asked to fill out a questionnaire about their symptoms, they responded as follows:

Physical Changes [1]

- 34% abdominal bloating
- 33% sore breasts
- 30% lower abdominal pain
- 29% backaches
- 26% uterine cramping
- 26% headaches
- 13% bloating and weight gain

Psychological/Emotional Changes

- 42% irritability
- 29% increased tension
- 27% depression
- 25% mood swings
- 16% unhappiness
- 13% shakiness
- 11% feelings of losing control

In 1938, McCance, Luff, and Widdowson studied irritability in relation to the menstrual cycle. They found a greater incidence of irritability premenstrually on Days 25 to 28, and menstrually on Days 1 to 3 than at any other time in the cycle. The next highest incidence was on Day 15, during ovulation. [2]

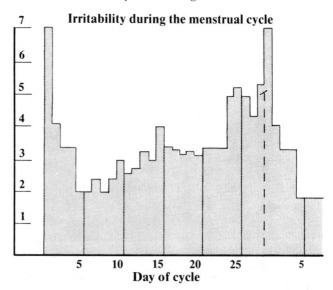

Irritability during the menstrual cycle

Day of cycle

Another group of researchers looked at employee absenteeism and found the highest incidence during menstruation, Days 1 to 4, and the next highest incidence on Days 13 to 16 (ovulation), and Days 25 to 28, during the premenstrual time.[3]

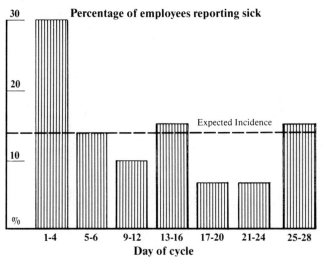

In a study of 174 hospital admissions, the *Proceedings of the Royal Society of Medicine* reported a significant increase in women admitted to hospitals during the premenstrual time, Days 25 to 28, and menstrually, during days 1 to 4.[4]

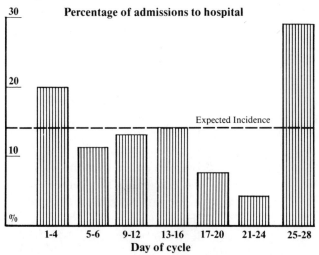

Tonks, Rack and Rose (1968) investigated suicide attempts during the menstrual cycle and found an unusually high incidence, above the expected rate, during the premenstrual time.[5]

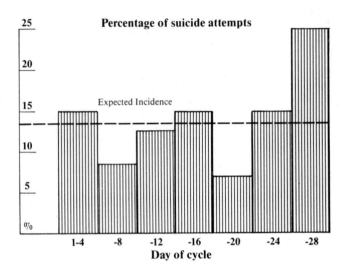

Percentage of suicide attempts

Expected Incidence

Day of cycle

WHO HAS PMS?

Premenstrual syndrome affects more women than most people realize. Eighty percent of all women have a problem with PMS at some time during their lives. For 10 percent of these women, the problems are disabling, severely affecting emotional stability, relationships, family life and careers. For that 10 percent, PMS can be a disease that destroys what would otherwise have been a normally productive, satisfying existence. It is the cause of much misery for the woman who has PMS, as well as for her friends and family.

According to Katharina Dalton, a British doctor whose pioneering work in the 1970s first alerted the medical community and then the world at large to the realities of premenstrual syndrome, 40 percent of women have premenstrual syndrome at any given point in time. That is, nearly half of the women you know have some degree of premenstrual problems every month.

Dalton found that PMS sufferers are most frequently in their thirties, and that a connection exists between PMS and hypertension in pregnancy, postpartum depression, and periods of stress. A tendency to PMS can be inherited. It has also been noted that women with PMS have a noticeable difficulty tolerating oral contraceptives.

Hysterectomy does not preclude PMS. Dalton notes that in one series of 34 women who had hysterectomies for non-malignant conditions, as many as 74 percent were later subject to "cyclically recurrent headaches," a common indication of PMS when it occurs on a monthly basis. Adolescents can have PMS, too, although it is often subtle, its symptoms mistakenly blamed on adolescent "behavior problems," "unsuitable friends," or "poor study habits."

2

THE
BASICS

Premenstrual syndrome is the subject of an exciting new field of research: that of the role of prostaglandins. Science is still at the early stages of discovering the Whys, Hows, and Whats of PMS and its relation to prostaglandins. Great progress has been made, however, in the last twenty years, and we can now successfully treat 90 percent of PMS cases.

THE CYCLE

To understand what happens to your body during the *pre*menstrual time, it helps to understand the full menstrual cycle and some of the changes that occur every month.

Day 1

This is the day on which menstruation begins, usually about 28 days after the beginning of the last month's menstruation. Not everyone has a 28-day cycle, however, and your Day 1 may be anywhere from 21 to 35 days after your last period began. It is on Day 1 that you produce the least amount of hormones in your entire month-long cycle. Day 1 also signals the beginning of production of one of these hormones—estrogen. From Day 1 until Day 15, you will be producing increasing amounts of estrogen, which makes the uterine lining grow, thicken and form glands that can provide nourishment for a fertilized egg.

Day 15 Day 15 is usually the time for ovulation. This is when an egg is released from the ovaries, and you begin producing another hormone—progesterone—as well as estrogen. Progesterone-stimulated glands in the uterus begin secreting nourishing substances and increase the blood supply in the uterus. Both progesterone and estrogen production will be high from now until the next Day 1, when they will make a dramatic dive down to nearly zero.

During the initial phases of the cycle, the uterus is building up an inner lining, or endometrium, that will be able to support and nourish a fertilized egg. When there is no fertilized egg, a series of events takes place that culminate in menstruation. First, estrogen and progesterone production virtually stop. Without these two hormones, the endometrium wall that lines the uterus begins to break away or "slough off." The uterine muscle contracts, which is felt as cramping. Contractions are brought on by a class of substances known as prostaglandins. This is menstruation, the beginning, or Day 1, of a new cycle.

BIO-CHEMICAL STRESS When your body is under biochemical stress, as it is during the premenstrual phase, it needs the B vitamins, also known as the "energy vitamins." Often, however, a craving for B vitamins gets confused with a craving for sugar, and instead of providing the B vitamins that we need, we give ourselves some sugar—a candy bar, for instance. It feels great, satisfying—just what we needed. But the satisfaction only lasts for a little while. Imperceptibly, we start to feel tired, to need another fix of sugar. Our insulin level has increased in order to handle the sugar, and we process and metabolize the sugar, but we have not gotten the vitamins and nutrients that we really needed. Again we crave these,

Day 1
Menstruation begins
No estrogen
No progesterone
Lining sloughs off

Estrogen and progesterone
production take a downward
dive; the uterine lining is
left with inadequate nutrients to
support its development
and growth

Estrogen production
builds up
uterine lining

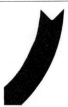

Day 15 (approximately)
Ovulation occurs when estrogen level in blood is high
Estrogen production continues
Progesterone production begins

and the cylce repeats itself as we eat sugar, our insulin levels rise, the sugar gets processed, we experience a "crash," and think we need more sugar.

Food cravings are often exaggerated in premenstrual syndrome. We're not certain why this happens, metabolically, but it is these food cravings that further add to our evidence that premenstrual syndrome is, in large part, a dietary problem.

It is biochemical stress that determines how much chemical coping is necessary for metabolism to work properly. There are many sources of what we call biochemical stress—from a broken arm or a bout with infection to a severe allergic reaction or a high fever, a heart condition or a prostaglandin problem. Under some circumstances we can deal with biochemical stresses that, under other conditions, would be overwhelming.

To understand this, you will temporarily have to put aside your concept of stress. Don't think of emotional stress, the kind that we are most intimately aware of— the unpaid bills, or the child who is having disciplinary problems at school. The kinds of stress we're talking about, besides obvious physical stress, are air pollution, food pollution (there are thousands of chemicals used to flavor, color, preserve and otherwise alter the food we eat; chemicals to protect food from insects and molds; chemicals to protect the animals meat and poultry come from; lead emissions from cars that stick to crops), noise pollution, and eating habits that do not fulfill our nutritional needs.

One hundred years ago we consumed an average of 5 pounds (2.25 kg) of sugar a year. The average sugar consumption among North Americans today is reported to be 150 pounds (67.5 kg) a year. Just working through that amount of sugar, much of it hidden in breakfast cereals and frozen vegetables, would put stress on any normal body. What was the biggest killer a century ago? Tuberculosis, an infectious disease. Today, metabolic stress leading to cardiovascular disease, myocardial problems, strokes, and the stress of lifestyle illnesses are the biggest killers.

Our systems and capabilities for dealing with the increasing stress are inadequate and the situation is getting worse. Premenstrual syndrome, we believe, is just one of a group of related health problems that have emerged since the 1970s, when the second generation of people born into this highly industrialized, chemicalized society came of age. Hyperactivity in children, the explosion of allergies, especially environmental and food "sensitivities," and stress-related diseases such as heart failure, are symptoms of our bodies' failure to cope adequately with the biochemical environmental stresses of the 1980s.

3

THE PROSTAGLANDIN CONNECTION

Prostaglandins are hormone-like substances found in almost every cell of the body. They influence widely varied metabolic processes. Groups of prostaglandins are crucial to the regulation of the nonvoluntary muscle systems, such as the heart, blood vessels, lungs, intestines, and uterus. While the prostaglandins vary in their specific effects, much of their influence depends not only on their amounts, but on their ratios —the ratio of one type of prostaglandin to another in any particular organ of the body. It is often the balance and combinations of prostaglandins that determine how well an organ is functioning.

Uterine contractions are mostly controlled by prostaglandins in what are called the E and F series. Prostaglandin F has been shown to cause contractions of the uterus; it is F that causes cramps during menstruation and childbirth—both of which are contractions of the uterus. Injections of prostaglandin F are used to induce spontaneous abortions.

Prostaglandin E-1 is the one we are most concerned with because of its central role in the female reproductive cycle. E-1 works in at least the following ways: as a vasodilator (opening up the blood vessels); as an inhibitor of thrombosis; as a controller of blood pressure; as a regulator of the immune system; as a powerful anti-inflammatory agent; as a defense against abnormal cell proliferation; and as an insulin regulator.

Prostaglandins were discovered in the early 1930s, when Ulf S. von Euler, a Swedish doctor, and other investigators reported that human semen and extracts of sheep seminal glands caused contractions of smooth muscle samples. They called the substances causing the contractions *prostaglandins* after the prostate gland where they were thought to originate.

Then, in the late 1940s, Sune K. Bergstrom, also a Swedish M.D., began to collaborate with von Euler. Bergstrom found that the prostaglandins were derived from fatty acids. In 1957, he isolated two prostaglandins, subsequently called PGE-1 and PGF-1a. That year, it was found that prostaglandins were present in menstrual fluid.

For their pioneering work, the 1982 Nobel Prize in Physiology or Medicine was awarded to Bergstrom and his research assistant, Bengt I. Samuelsson, also of Sweden, along with John R. Vane from the Wellcome Research Foundation in England. In 1971, Vane's research student, Jim Willis, showed that aspirin and other drugs called NSAIDS (non-steroidal anti-inflammatory drugs) work by blocking the major step in the body's synthesis of prostaglandins. Since then, the prostaglandins have become a hot topic for researchers; they are the subject of numerous papers and reports. Prostaglandins have been found to influence nearly every organ and function of the body.

The precise structure of two series of prostaglandins was discovered in 1962, and seven specific types of prostaglandins were identified. Like the vitamins, these were given letter names: E, F, A, B, C and D.

In 1973, David Horrobin, a physician specializing in nutrition and chronic health problems, unintentionally discovered that prostaglandins are related to premenstrual syndrome. At the time he was researching the effects of prolactin, a pituitary hormone that helps to regulate progesterone production and to stimulate the mammary glands.

During the course of his research he injected himself with prolactin on several occasions. "I became what can only be described as premenstrual," says Horrobin. "I swelled up, felt irritable, bloated, depressed, fed up. My experience was remarkably similar to what women describe during the premenstrual phase."

Following up this remarkable discovery with lab work, Horrobin found that essential fatty acids are converted in the body into prostaglandin E-1, the prostaglandin that has beneficial effects during the premenstrual time. He also found that E-1 dampens the undesirable effects of prolactin.

THE ESSENTIAL FATTY ACID CONVERSION

The prostaglandins are made from substances called *essential fatty acids*, which are the polyunsaturated fats that we've heard so much about in relation to heart disease. Our bodies cannot manufacture the essential fatty acids; like minerals, vitamins and the essential amino acids, they must be provided from outside sources. One of the most important essential fatty acids, converted in the body into prostaglandin E-1, is linoleic acid (LA). The conversion pathway includes gamma-linolenic acid (GLA), dihomogamma-linolenic acid, and finally, prostaglandin E-1.

The conversion process from linoleic acid, which we get from dietary sources, to prostaglandin E-1 requires co-factors—nutrients that "grease" the system and provide vital elements. These co-factors are vitamin B6 (pyridoxine), zinc, niacin, vitamin C (ascorbic acid), and magnesium. (See the chart on the next page.)

Linoleic acid, the essential fatty acid necessary for the manufacture of prostaglandin E-1 is normally found in certain vegetable oils, including safflower and sunflower oil. It is not present in substantial quantities in other oils (such as olive, palm, or coconut oil), and it may be rendered useless when vegetable oils are processed. Heat from cooking procedures, such as deep frying, can destroy the effectiveness of the linoleic acid. Hydrogenation, which is used to make margarines, is one step worse than useless: margarine not only destroys the linoleic acid of the natural oils, but it blocks other essential fatty acids from being used.

When linoleic acid obtained from the diet is converted to gammalinolenic acid, the rest of the process unfolds and progresses with the final result of prostaglandin E-1. Sometimes, however, our bodies are not able to convert the linoleic acid of our foods into gammalinolenic acid. Some of the problems preventing this conversion have been found to include: a diet rich in saturated fats or processed vegetable oils such as margarine (both of which compete with the essential fatty acids); moderate to high consumption of alcoholic beverages; diabetes; the aging process; vitamin and/or mineral deficiencies (especially of the B vitamins, vitamin C, zinc, and magnesium); viral infections; radiation; and cancer.

Those of us who are unable to synthesize prostaglandins in the right amounts and in the right proportions develop a wide variety of problems—especially in the reproductive, cardiovascular, dermatological and immune systems. Premenstrual syndrome is one of the problems that often develops from a lack of balanced prostaglandins.

THE EFA CHAIN

foods
containing
essential
fatty acids
(polyunsaturates)

cis-linoleic
acid

evening primrose oil
bypasses this
block without
dietary adjustments

conversion blocked
by cholesterol,
saturated fats,
processed vegetable oils,
alcohol, aging, diabetes,
zinc deficiency
and viral infections.

human milk
and evening primrose
oil

gammalinolenic
acid

pyridoxine probably
necessary for
conversion

human milk

dihomogamma-
linolenic acid

zinc, niacin,
ascorbic acid
necessary for
conversion

see text for
functions

prostaglandin
E1

Gammalinolenic acid is present in usable form and sufficient quantity in very few substances. As mentioned earlier in the book, to date we know of only two sources: human breast milk and evening primrose seed oil. (In small quantities, insufficient for practical use, it is also present in borage, an annual herb grown in temperate climates.) Thus, prostaglandin E-1 can be produced directly from the gammalinolenic acid provided by the evening primrose seed oil (or human breast milk), as long as the various co-factors are also supplied.

Our clinical reseach experience has shown that when there is an increase in prostaglandin E-1—that is, when we are provided the means to produce prostaglandin E-1—there is a significant reduction in premenstrual syndrome problems. With a nutritional approach alone, we have had a 70 percent success rate with premenstrual syndrome.

4

THE TRAGEDY OF PMS

Sometime in early 1982, a woman came into an emergency center. The staff person who saw her was familiar with premenstrual syndrome and saw that Meg C. had classic symptoms recurring like clockwork every month just before her period. Although Meg's problems had the appearance of being emotional/psychological, he realized that they were, in fact, premenstrual.

Meg herself had realized the cyclical nature of her upsets for several years, but had been unable to find anyone who believed her. When she came to us, she had charted her mood swings and outbursts over a period of six months and could thus show that the explosions of temper occurred consistently one week before the onset of her period.

Everything would go along fine, she explained, and she would feel generally happy and contented for three weeks at a time. Then, everything would "fall apart." She would feel miserable, and find herself furious over minor details, subject to temper tantrums, forgetful of important details of everyday life—such as paying bills *and* keeping money in the checking account. She said it was as if she were a different person.

We gave Meg vitamin B$_6$, vitamin C and vitamin B-complex, and put her on a well balanced nutrient program with evening primrose oil to provide gammalinolenic acid. Meg's problems were brought well under control within three months. She eventually moved to another state, but a year or so later, she called again, in tears.

"Thank goodness you're there," she said, and launched into a tale of how she'd felt so good that she had stopped taking the nutrients. She had moved to Kansas for a new job, but while there had begun to experience the same kinds of problems as before, quite severely. The temper tantrums and the inability to cope with everyday details had all returned. She was crying on the phone as she explained crisis days where everything seemed to dissolve into complete disaster for her. She'd gone to an internist, she said, and had explained to him that hers was a simple problem of premenstrual syndrome.

"No, you don't have PMS," the doctor informed her.

"But I do," Meg insisted, and began to describe her history of PMS symptoms prior to diagnosis, and the syndrome's successful treatment. The doctor, however, refused to take her seriously.

"You can't have PMS," he said, "because your symptoms are too intense for PMS." He looked at her sympathetically. "PMS is just not as bad as this. You need professional help. You need to see a psychiatrist if you want to get better. If you don't want to get better, of course, you don't have to . . ." His voice trailed off meaningfully, but Meg had gotten the message: You have psychological problems, and if you don't go to a psychiatrist, you don't really want help.

Meg was given a referral to a psychiatrist and prescriptions for antidepressants and diuretics. These three are the classic cure for "female problems."

Dear Dr. Lombard:

I am 36 years old and in excellent health, except that I have been troubled for the last four or five years by the symptoms of breast tenderness, fluid retention, headaches, irritability and anxiety, which usually begin approximately two weeks before my period. I have told my doctor, but he simply tells me to limit my salt.

Depression is also a problem during this time, as is an inability to consume alcoholic beverages.

Any help you can be with this matter will be greatly appreciated.

Dear Sir/Madame:

I feel I may be suffering from premenstrual syndrome or food allergies. I have been to doctors during this three-year misery, but none have done any tests. They just prescribe tranquillizers, which I refuse to take . . .

Dear Dr. Nazzaro and Dr. Lombard:

Thank you! I'm not crazy after all! And it's not "all in my head."

Your workshop and your research regarding PMS has made all the difference in my life and my relationships with others, particularly my family. Prior to attending the workshops, I manifested all of the classic PMS symptoms—mood swings, depression, anxiety, headache, etc. I can safely say that all symptoms have responded to your suggested nutritional supplements by 80 to 100 percent. And my menstrual cycle has regulated itself, with decreased bleeding and no intermittent spotting, both of which were problems before.

Again, many thanks for offering these workshops. But most importantly, thanks for helping me overcome PMS.

Dear Dr. Nazzaro:

Please send me any information you have available concerning premenstrual syndrome and its treatment. I could hardly believe it when I read an article about you and premenstrual syndrome, because that must be what is wrong with me.

I have gone to my family practitioner at least five times in the last few years, telling him that I go through terrible mood swings for about a week and a half, just before my period starts every month. I get really crazy and I scare myself as well as my loved ones, and sometimes even get to the point where I hurt myself (I do not hurt them). Last time, I just stopped myself from throwing a lovely procelain sugar bowl—an heirloom passed down from my great-grandmother— across the room over some insignificant matter.

But this sort of thing only happens during the "premenstrual" time. The rest of the month I am a different person; calm, relaxed, generally easy-going and happy. I do not feel that I'm schizophrenic.

My family doctor says to take tranquillizers and/or go to a psychiatrist. I don't want to take tranquillizers because I don't want to rely on heavy drugs, *and I can't really afford to see a psychiatrist. I keep asking him for a blood test or something, because I really feel like there's a chemical change that happens to me every month. But he always says there is nothing that can be done about it except tranquillizers and psychiatrists.*

Anyway, I'd appreciate any information you can give me. Thank you very much, in advance.

Dear Dr. Lombard and Dr. Nazzaro:

I need your help! My 14-year-old daughter and myself suffer from PMS of varying degrees.

Our cycles are within hours of each other, and needless to say, we hate each other. My husband and our other two children would like to leave home.

We are now in family counselling, and recently my daughter attempted suicide. Fortunately, she is still in good health—except for PMS. But we have not been able to locate any physician knowledgeable in PMS treatment. Is it at all possible for you to send me information about the nutrition program? If you feel you cannot help from such a distance, please send recommendations. Maybe something one of our doctors here could read. My marriage is in danger and I can't seem to help myself—or my daughter.

Please help us.

These are typical of the letters we have received from all over the country from women looking for treatment for PMS. Why is it that so many women are prescribed drugs and diuretics, or sent to psychiatrists when their problems are not emotional, not a simple matter of water retention, and not psychological? Why is it that the typical (although there are a growing number of exceptions) family practitioner or gynecologist continues to respond to premenstrual complaints with patronizing phrases and empty talk about "getting used to it"? Why do so many doctors still react with disbelief when told that premenstrual syndrome is a medical problem—with a medical solution?

A patient of ours recently told us of this conversation with her father, a general practitioner:

"I'm seeing a doctor who is going to help me with premenstrual syndrome, Dad. Are you familiar with premenstrual syndrome? Remember how when I was a teenager living at home I always got so moody right before my periods, and how I bloated up, and got irritable and depressed? That's typical of PMS, and they are realizing that it can be treated."

"What are you talking about?" asked her father. "PMS? That's how women have *always* felt, there's nothing unusual in what you're saying. What do you mean, a *medical condition*? That's just how it is for women. Why are you making a fuss over it?"

The mother, overhearing the conversation, had this to add: "Take some tranquillizers when you feel that way dear. That's how we women get through it. That's how we've always gotten through it. Remember Aunt Edith? She always took tranquillizers before her period. Things were very bad for her. How did you think we women get through life?"

The underlying reason for this prolonged ignorance on the part of our doctors is that it often takes five to ten years before information filters down from the research labs to the doctors' offices. The practitioners tend to be so busy with their patients that they can't keep abreast of the plethora of new information constantly spewing from the universities and research labs. They receive dozens of medical journals every month, they go to as many lectures concerning new findings and treatment procedures as they can, they talk to "detail men" from the pharmaceutical firms, who brief them on the latest in drugs and equipment. Findings that are not promoted by the media or the drug companies tend to get drowned out in the sea of information.

It is not so much doctors' resistance to changing their habitual diagnoses or to learning about new treatments for such problems as it is the system they are locked into; a system in which, for example, nutrition is not a priority. Like all people, doctors usually continue in the paths they were taught; it's not easy to learn alternative approaches. They look for explanations they are familiar with, explanations that are acceptable. They search on, often valiantly if mistakenly, until they find a "reasonable" explanation.

Research testing of treatment for premenstrual syndrome, as well as studies of the disease itself, are currently underway. As more and more doctors become aware of PMS as a medical condition, and as research findings are published, it is becoming recognized in doctors' offices everywhere. Because the research is being conducted in many different countries, it adds several more years onto the filtration process from the labs to the journals to the doctors. Medical consumers who want the best possible health care will have to enter into partnerships with their doctors, to speed up the acceptance and use of valid, useful and safe medical discoveries—including treatment for PMS.

In addition, however, doctors tend to lag behind on problems like PMS because if there is no clinical or lab test for a medical condition it tends not to "exist" in the eyes of the medical profession. What we mean is that if there is no test for an illness or a condition, then it cannot be definitively diagnosed. Without a diagnosis, how can it be treated? Put differently, if there is no way to test for something, it cannot be named, and in the root sense of the word *named*, it then has no reality or power.

Here is one scenario of what may happen when a woman goes into a doctor's office and says, "I'm irritable, I'm depressed, I'm snappish, I'm jumpy." That combination of symptoms is automatically filed mentally under *P* for *psychiatric* by the doctor. The woman is then sent to a psychiatrist or some other mental health professional.

Perhaps you can imagine how ridiculous this feels a few years later when the healthcare provider learns about premenstrual syndrome. We know how depressing and ridiculous it feels because we were there, using psychopharmacology and psychiatry for women who had premenstrual syndrome. It is painful to think back on those women who were told they were emotionally disturbed when what they really had was a physical problem—premenstrual syndrome.

PSYCHIATRIC TREATMENT

Right now—this very day, this very minute—there are women who are seeing psychiatrists for PMS, digging very hard into their problems from a psychological point of view in the vain hope of curing biochemical imbalances. They are searching their childhood in a fruitless effort to find a psychological cause for a physical affliction.

Psychiatry is a common treatment for PMS and has been for many years. Talking therapy, tranquillizers, anti-depressants, diuretics, and mood elevators are matter-of-course for premenstrual syndrome problems in a psychiatric setting.

But think of it. Antidepressants work on specific neurotransmitters in the brain. They can offset some of the effects of PMS, but they do not help the syndrome itself. Nor do they help with any of the other manifestations of PMS, such as bloating, lethargy, and food cravings. Mood elevators and antidepressants require three to six weeks to take effect. Most women taking them for PMS end up relying on them for extended periods, perhaps for years. Diuretics also treat only one aspect of the symptom. They are good for helping to restore fluid balance, but they don't begin to tackle the other problems of PMS.

Here is a typical scenario. A woman knows that she is "just not doing well." So she goes to her general practitioner or family doctor.

"Doctor," she says, "I don't really know what the problem is, and I don't really know what you can do for me. The thing is, I feel terrible sometimes. And sometimes, though, I'm okay. Something is wrong, doctor, but I just don't know what it is. I get feeling so down, and it seems as if everything is going wrong, everything is awful, and then it's all okay again. But then it gets bad a few weeks later."

Maybe the woman is able to be somewhat more specific.

"I don't know, Doctor," she continues, "I just keep on getting these symptoms, where I get headachy and I'm tired. Exhausted. Everything feels like it's too much for me. I get real moody. I'm hungry all of the time, and I feel bloated. Sometimes I have to put on clothes that are a size larger, or I wear sweatpants because they have an elastic waistband. I don't know what is going on with me. Then, I'll be okay—but it keeps coming back. It seems like it's been this way for a long time and I'm really tired of it, and I need help. Do you know what's wrong with me? Can you help me please?"

The woman is often anxious and imagines all sorts of things that might be wrong. The doctor, a trained medical professional, goes on a search, a medical hunt to uncover the problem. He runs all of the standard medical tests. The tests themselves can be a frightening experience, and waiting for results can add to the already high level of anxiety. The process can drag on for months and can be a gruelling one. Then, the day dawns when all of the tests have come back and they are all normal—every one of them. The doctor has run all the tests he thinks are reasonably appropriate, but he hasn't been able to uncover the problem. He can't think of any more tests that would make sense, and he doesn't want to lead the patient on.

What is left? "It must be emotional." Emotional origin is a "reasonable" diagnosis and there are ways to treat such problems, mostly through medication and psychotherapy. The woman has been feeling "off balance" periodically for the last several years because of her extreme irritability. By now, after all of this medical hunting, after all of these raised eyebrows and with this medical conclusion, she believes that she does need psychiatric help. Indeed, psychiatric help will be of great comfort for her. After the long struggle to get help for her problems, it will feel good to have a sympathetic ear. Maybe she does have a few emotional imperfections, anyway.

The psychiatrist, of course, is very understanding and non-judgmental. The psychiatrist has an intuitive sense about the kind of pain this woman is in. The woman begins to feel better, going to the psychiatrist once, twice, maybe three times a week and talking it all out. She still has PMS, but she also has an outlet. She feels that it is better than nothing at all, and it is.

The other route to the psychiatrist's couch is via the gynecologist.

"I have terrible cramps, Doctor," complains our prototype. "They come every month, just before my period.

I feel terrible. I get rundown and sick all the time. I don't know what to do."

The woman is given a prostaglandin inhibitor such as Motrin, Ponstel, or aspirin, and it may take care of her cramps—but it does not handle the other problems.

Sympathy, understanding, a pat on the back, and a pep talk follow. The woman returns home feeling chastised and determined to "learn to live with it." She should get more control over her feelings, the gynecologist said. Or she should learn how to express herself better, or earlier. The next month, when she begins to feel the bloating and tension coming on, she thinks about how she should be learning to live with it. "That's just part of being a woman," she tells herself again, repeating her doctor's admonitions. "I'll just have to learn to live with it."

After a few cycles, however, most women realize that they cannot simply learn to live with it. It isn't like a cold, it isn't like a broken arm. It is more like a migraine headache, or a heart attack, or some other stress-related problem. They can't live with it and it is upsetting their lives, both at work and at home. Their kids won't talk to them for a week at a time. Their husbands or friends are becoming defensive and unsympathetic. Their co-workers avoid them.

Typically, these women go back to the gynecologist's office and push for a diagnosis and treatment. Finally, the doctor makes a decision.

"Okay," he says. "You should see a psychiatrist. This is purely emotional. I can find no physical reason for you to be feeling this way."

Off to the psychiatrist's office goes our woman, now embarked on a much different course than would have been considered had her doctor been familiar with the rudiments of premenstrual syndrome and its medical basis.

There is yet another route to the psychiatrist's couch. A woman has a friend with similar problems who is seeing a psychiatrist. This friend advises her to do the same. She works out some of her underlying psychiatric problems, but she is still plagued by PMS.

Thus, the psychiatric route is the most common avenue of PMS treatment. Popular drugs prescribed by psychiatrists or other doctors include Valium, Librium, Elavil, Tofranil, and Mellaril. At best they usually help one or two symptoms of the PMS problem and can be associated with side effects.

So, the usual response of doctors when a woman complains of PMS symptoms is that there is nothing at all wrong with her and that her symptoms are the result of emotional/psychological problems; or that it is part of being a woman.

OTHER TREATMENT APPROACHES

Prostaglandin imbalance and its correction through the use of a nutritional approach is not the only current treatment for premenstrual syndrome available today. There are several other methods that have been introduced to those suffering from PMS. They include medications to reduce levels of certain hormones plus treatments that augment other hormones. We'd like to take a moment to go over some of these treatment methods so you can have an idea of what's available.

Progesterone

The treatment for PMS that has received the most publicity in the media is that of progesterone supplementation. This is in part because the work of PMS pioneer Katharina Dalton is based on this method.

The basic theory behind progesterone supplementation stems from the idea that there is a faulty progesterone feedback pathway in the biochemical relationships between the hypothalamus, pituitary gland, uterus and ovaries—resulting in a deficiency of progesterone. The deficiency is caused by either a lack of production of progesterone, or the interference of metabolism of progesterone by other hormones. Prolactin appears to be the hormone most responsible for this interference.

The treatment of PMS based on this theory depends on two areas: 1) supplementing with progesterone; and 2) stopping the interference in the production by the use of the prolactin inhibitor, bromocryptine.

The Use of Progesterone

There are several ways to supplement progesterone. Dyprogesterone is an oral tablet form of progesterone that is generally taken during the last half of the cycle. Progesterone is also found in suppository form and this seems to be the form most often used. These are generally used for seven to fourteen days during the last half of the menstrual cycle. Norethisterone is a synthetic that is very close to natural progesterone, but seems to be associated with a greater likelihood of side effects.

There has been a lot of controversy associated with the use of progesterone. There are indications that progesterone does not work as well as was initially expected in handling PMS symptoms and the long term effects of supplementing with progesterone are not certain, although there appear to be no ill effects. In addition, many women who have used progesterone supplementation have reported a variety of side effects. In her recently published book, *The Premenstrual Syndrome*, Caroline Mozelle notes that unwanted side effects of progesterone can include depression, migraine-like headaches, visual disturbances, blood clotting, raised blood pressure, and jaundice. It is important, however, to note that not all women get these side effects, and some women have reported freedom from their symptoms with the use of progesterone.

Our program does not include the use of progesterone supplementation. We have found little reason to use it with our patients. The majority of our patients respond well to the nutritional program or fall into one of the problem categories we will be describing later in this book (chapter 7).

Prolactin Inhibition

Another method associated with the treatment of PMS is the use of the prolactin inhibitor, bromocryptine. Prolactin is a hormone that is produced in the pituitary gland. When most women think of prolactin they think of the production of breast milk, but prolactin has also been shown to play a role in symptoms associated with PMS.

Generally, when a prolactin excess is suspected, the best way to find out if prolactin is playing a role in a PMS problem is to take a prolactin test. This is a blood test, which your physician can order, that will show the level of prolactin being produced. If this is higher than the normal range, then it is possible that bringing the level down can relieve some of the PMS symptoms. Bromocryptine is a medication used specifically to reduce the level of prolactin. It is important to stress that the use of bromocryptine is not specifically a treatment for PMS, but may be an aid that your physician will consider. The trade name for bromocryptine is Parlodel and it comes in 2.5 mg and 10 mg tablets. When administered, it is usually given gradually, starting with a small dose and then working up to a higher one. Some women report side effects associated with the use of bromocryptine. Among the most noted are dizziness, nausea, vomiting, headache, and constipation.

We have found the use of bromocryptine helpful with women who have higher than normal levels of prolactin and, when indicated, will use the medication along with the nutrient program for optimum results.

Diuretics

Another common treatment approach is to prescribe diuretics (medications that prevent the retention of excess fluid in the body tissues). This stems from water retention being a common symptom of PMS. Generally, a medication such as chlorothiazide (trade name Diuril) or hydrochlorothiazide (Hydrodiuril) is prescribed. These medications are specific to water retention and cannot help the other symptoms of PMS. In addition, side effects such as headaches, dizziness, and a dry mouth can be associated with the use of diuretics.

OTHER NUTRI— TIONAL APPROACHES

There are several other nutritional approaches available. Vitamin B_6, for example, has been gaining prominence in the area of PMS symptom relief. It is our feeling that this vitamin has an important part in a nutritional regimen and that it plays an important role in helping to alleviate specific symptoms of PMS. However, it is also our feeling that a better approach would be to incorporate the use of B_6 into a total program of nutritional support. The use of certain nutrients without the support of others can create its own specific problems. The B vitamins often work in concert with each other. When you supplement one in higher amounts without considering the others, an imbalance of certain B vitamins may result, along with the loss of optimum efficiency.

OTHER REMEDIES

The psychiatric route is not the only response to women who have PMS. Another common response is "Have a baby."

We do not consider this to be an appropriate treatment for PMS; it is not effective. While it is true that a few women with PMS have been known to feel better after giving birth, it is even more common for them to become premenstrual *after* pregnancy and childbirth when they were not premenstrual prior to it. Often, PMS becomes worse and worse with each successive pregnancy.

Alcohol

Alcohol is another traditional "remedy." Grandma used to recommend alcohol for cramps during menstruation, as well as for problems the week or so before it. As a central nervous system depressant, alcohol dulls the feelings and relaxes a person for a short period of time. However, it does not help the syndrome, and it depletes necessary nutrients. If a woman has a problem with alcoholism, it is an especially dangerous time because the effects of each drink are heightened. It is also a time when women with drinking problems tend to have bouts of heavy drinking, partly as a result of distress and depression, and partly because of the biochemical demands of their addiction.

Baths

Grandma also used to favor long soaks in a hot tub. Yes, this delightful home remedy has merit for helping to alleviate immediate symptoms, and it is a lovely thing to do. We highly recommend relaxation in general, but it will not even begin to handle the real problems of PMS.

Hysterectomy

The worst treatment of all for PMS is hysterectomy. The use of hysterectomy to treat premenstrual syndrome is a medical tragedy, yet it continues to happen. Typically, a woman visits her doctor month after month in severe pain. After the doctor has taken all of the tests he can think of that might lead to a diagnosis and is still unable to uncover the roots of the problem, he may recommend that she undergo exploratory surgery. This happens especially when the patient insists that her problem is not psychological in origin, but is, instead, "real." Generally, the idea behind this exploratory surgery is to discover if endometriosis, characterized by cysts and adhesions, may be causing the premenstrual difficulties. Sometimes what happens is that the surgeon performs a hysterectomy; the reasoning being "if we take everything out, you won't be bothered anymore."

This reasoning, however, is flawed. Hysterectomy is not only major surgery that changes the hormonal system for life (especially if the ovaries are removed), but, in fact, hysterectomy can make PMS worse. Especially if her ovaries have been left intact, a woman who has had a hysterectomy may still find herself subject to cyclical changes. Even without her period, she may have "premenstrual syndrome," with symptoms that recur every month. Her ovaries continue to produce cyclical changes in hormone levels, but these are not obvious because the uterus has been removed.

Take the case of Emily, a 45-year-old woman who has had severe PMS since puberty. She tried progesterone therapy, aspirin, giving up food that contains caffeine—including coffee, chocolate, tea, colas, and various medications. She limited her salt intake. She took diuretics. She went in for counselling. Finally, however, her premenstrual problems became so difficult that her doctor advised her to have a complete hysterectomy.

While lying in the hospital bed the day after the operation, Emily opened a women's magazine to an article describing premenstrual syndrome, and the high success rate of the nutritional approach. She was devastated. Moreover, she soon discovered that she was still premenstrual.

Months after the hysterectomy, she found that her symptoms were nearly as bad as they had been before the operation. She came to our office and we did a full evaluation of her, finding that she had severe allergies and a probable prostaglandin E-1 problem. Emily used to say, "If I hadn't had the hysterectomy, if I was still getting my period, then *this* would be my premenstrual week. I'm bloating up. I feel awful. I've been having bad mood swings, . . ." She has been able to bring the premenstrual problem under control through dietary means, and she has been treating herself for her allergies.

5

THE SOLUTION

The basis of our evaluation—and the basis of doing your own evaluation—is trust. You'll just have to believe in yourself and in your analysis of how you feel. After all, why shouldn't you believe yourself? You are not out to trick yourself, so forget it when your friends or your husband or even your doctor tells you that you are "imagining" something or "making a big deal out of nothing." Forget the neighbor or the mother-in-law who says you are just babying yourself and that you'd be fine if you would just "join the garden club," "get a job," "get involved with the PTA," etc. "You'd feel fine," says your sister, "if you'd put yourself out for other people a little more or had a more active social life." People may tell you that you'd feel fine, if you didn't work so hard, or if you worked a little harder, or if you didn't worry so much. Even your best friend may say, "I never had such problems—but even if I did, I wouldn't make such a fuss over it. I would just get on with my life."

The problem is, it's hard or even impossible to get on with your life when you have PMS. Most women with PMS find that it plays a major role in their lives and that it affects them not only during the premenstrual weeks, but during the rest of the month, too, when they tend to expend a great deal of energy trying to make up for things that they did or said—or didn't do or say—during their pre-time. You need to face the problem—and treat it, because it will not get better by itself.

Don't worry about what other people think. If you know you have a problem, get it taken care of. Believing in yourself is the first step. For many women, it is the most difficult one.

To evaluate whether a woman coming to our office has PMS, we first try to get a sense of her immediate problems. Are the symptoms typical of PMS? Do they appear 2 to 14 days before her period? Do they disappear or recede significantly when she gets her period? If so, then she is likely to have PMS.

We next take a full personal history, including events from early childhood, both medical and non-medical. One of the specifics we listen for is the use of antibiotics. This is because heavy, prolonged, or repeated antibiotic use sets the stage for a common complicating factor of premenstrual syndrome called *intestinal yeast overgrowth*. An intestinal yeast overgrowth, or *Candida albicans*, can exacerbate premenstrual problems or it can be mistaken for premenstrual syndrome.

In addition to the early childhood history and the history of antibiotics use, we learn about when the woman had her first period and the kinds of symptoms she had during her early years of menstruation. What about her adolescence in general? Did she have emotional problems? Problems at school? At home? Medical problems? Bone fractures? Did she participate in sports? What kinds of food did she eat regularly? Did she go on any weight-loss or weight-gain diets? Did she take birth control pills? Was she fitted with an intrauterine device (IUD)? How long did she use either of these methods of birth control? What symptoms or problems were associated with them? What method did she switch to and why? Has she ever been pregnant? Has she had any miscarriages or abortions? Did she give birth? (Birth control pills, the IUD, and pregnancy all provide a climate that is conducive to yeast overgrowth.)

When the facts are put together in logical sequence, the connections usually become apparent. Even without help from a physician, most women can put their clinical history together logically. For instance, in a typical interview we'll be told that the symptoms of mood swings and breast soreness began in a woman's early 20s. Then we'll hear that she began using birth control pills in her early 20s. "Did your symptoms begin *before* or *after* you began taking birth control pills?" we ask. Typically, the response is, "You know, I never had any symptoms until I started taking the pill." This is the way someone trying to see her medical patterns should review her medical history. Chart your history, year by year, and try to make the connections that will enable you to see the entire picture.

We also take a family history and focus special attention on whether premenstrual problems run in the family. Because of the connection between prostaglandin imbalance and hyperactivity in young children, especially boys, we also look for a family history of hyperactivity.

In addition, we want to know about cigarette smoking, the drug history, what nutrients or vitamins—if any— the patient has taken regularly (and what effects they had). We look into her past and present exercise habits, including why she chooses the exercises she does. We want to know what she eats and what her favorite foods are. We are finding that allergies are sometimes connected with premenstrual syndrome and can exacerbate the problem. What inhalants is she normally breathing? Gasoline vapors in cars or buses? Perfumes? Cleaning products, plastics, fabrics with formaldehyde? Which of these things, if any, is she aware of having reactions to? We ask about her bowel movements: Is she regular? Are her stools light or dark? Do they float or sink? Bowel problems are often related to yeast infections, PMS, or allergies, and also help to give an accurate idea of general health.

If we suspect an allergy factor, we take a complete history of sensitivity to chemicals, inhalants, and foods. We want to know about food cravings, headaches, and other symptoms, and when they occur in the menstrual cycle. (See the appendix at the back of the book for an allergy checklist.)

A physical examination is done, along with a complete blood count, blood chemistries, urinalysis, and possibly a thyroid test. One reason for these lab tests is to ascertain whether the thyroid is operating efficiently. Thyroid problems can be very tricky, and it is crucial to look into the possibility of thyroid malfunction.

Thyroid malfunction should always be considered before any course of vitamin supplementation begins. A simple pre-test is to take your axillary temperature for three mornings in a row. That is, hold a thermometer in the armpit for 10 minutes. If the temperature is below 97° F (36° C) for three days in a row, a thyroid problem may be present. Anyone whose axillary temperature is consistently below 97° should seek the help of a professional.

*Hyper*thyroidism (a thyroid that is too active) can make you feel irritable, depressed, and have more sweat and heat intolerance. More common is *hypo*thyroidism (a thyroid that is underactive), with sluggishness, depression, irritability, dry skin, cold intolerance, hoarseness, weight gain, and constipation. Either of these problems, however, can be confused with premenstrual syndrome. We caution that the thyroid is terribly difficult to be sure of without lab tests. Because it is intimately involved in the metabolic processes, the possibility that someone with severe premenstrual syndrome has the complicating factor of a thyroid problem must be considered.

We look for the following patterns, problems that commonly complicate or imitate premenstrual syndrome:

- problems with vaginal infections
- a history of taking oral contraceptives
- a history of heavy dosages of antibiotics, or frequent use of antibiotics.
- food or inhalant sensitivities
- the presence of symptoms not only during the premenstrual time but at other times of the month as well

If a woman has *not* had any of these problems, yet suffers from symptoms that fit the PMS description as outlined earlier, then we consider her to be manifesting PMS and we suggest a trial of supplements.

However, if we have a woman who, besides having all the usual symptoms of PMS, says that she doesn't feel well for the rest of the month either, that her symptoms simply get worse at her premenstrual time, that she never really feels that she has gotten back on top of things, and that she has additional problems such as constipation and/or diarrhea or other bowel and stomach problems; or a history of antibiotic usage; or she has been on birth control pills, *then* we consider the possibility that there is yeast in the intestinal tract that is exacerbating the premenstrual syndrome. A yeast overgrowth cannot be controlled through nutritional means alone. This condition requires other treatment, which we will detail later (in chapter 7).

If, in addition to the PMS symptoms, the woman also exhibits very low energy, gets noticeably sleepy after meals, gets headaches, or is affected by perfumes or gases, then we may suspect an allergy or "sensitivity" problem. This should be treated along with the premenstrual syndrome.

The bottom line for a PMS diagnosis is: *Do the symptoms return on a regular basis between 2 and 14 days before menstruation, and do they decrease significantly when menstruation begins?* With this pattern it is fairly simple to distinguish PMS from clinical depression as well, where symptoms usually exist throughout the entire month and where there is a good response to psychotropic medications and therapy.

If there is a clear-cut case of premenstrual syndrome—one that is not mediated by allergies, yeast, or other complications—we start the patient on a nutrient program immediately. The program is worked and reworked so that it is eventually geared specifically to her. One woman may experience depression and some bloating, while another may have breast soreness, irritability and migraine headaches. Each has a prostaglandin imbalance, but they will probably require different amounts of nutritional supplements to help their bodies produce the proper balance of prostaglandins for optimal relief.

Optimal relief, rather than average relief, is what we are looking for. It is what any individual should look for—and work to achieve. To accept anything less is to cheat yourself and those around you.

THE SELF-EVALUATION QUIZ

Now that you know the kind of information we look for, it's time for you to do a self-evaluation to determine if PMS is a problem for you. This questionnaire will also help you to organize your medical and symptom history to take to your physician.

The best way to fill out this questionnaire for maximum information is to go through it once and answer all the questions to which you immediately know the answer.

Then go through it again and mark any questions you will have to check with your physician or consult medical records about. Then leave it for a day or two. This will allow you to think about all the symptoms that you may have forgotten about. After a few days, go back to it and fill in any additional information you have remembered.

After you have completed the questionnaire, you will begin to have a better idea of what your symptoms are, when they occur, and how much they interfere with your day-to-day living patterns. Take this questionnaire with you when you go to see your doctor. It will save you time and will help to ensure that you both know all the facts.

PERSONAL HEALTH
and MENSTRUATION HISTORY

Name:_____

Birthdate: _____

Number of days in cycle:_____

List and describe any symptoms you have for either part of the month or all month long (consider duration and intensity):

_____

_____

_____

_____

_____

List the symptoms mentioned above that subside with the onset of your period:

_____

_____

_____

_____

How long have you had these symptoms? When did they first appear and have they gotten worse with time?

_____

_____

_____

_____

The symptoms that subside with your period or shortly thereafter are most likely PMS symptoms. The remaining symptoms will be categorized as *other*. During the remainder of this questionnaire, we will be indicating which set of symptoms we are asking about in each question. You may not be able to determine clearly the category you suspect for each symptom, but do the best you can.

GENERAL HEALTH and PRESENT PROBLEMS
Do you now get frequent colds or flu?

_____

_____

Do you have problems with your eyes? If yes, describe what the problems are and when they occur.

_____

_____

_____

Do you have problems with your ears? If yes, describe what the problems are and when they occur.
PMS: _____

_____

_____

Other:_____

_____

_____

Do you have problems with your nose (runny nose, post-nasal drip, etc.)?

PMS: _____

_____

_____

Other: _____

_____

_____

Do you have any cardiac problems (known heart problems, high blood pressure, occasional palpitations, etc.)? When and under what circumstances?
PMS: _____

_____

Other: _____

_____

_____

Do you have any lung or respiratory problems (infections, shortness of breath, asthma, etc.)?
PMS: _____

_____

Other: _____

_____

_____

Do you have any gastrointestinal problems (bloating, stomach aches, pain or burning)?
PMS: _____

_____

Other: _____

_____

_____

Do you have problems with constipation and/or diarrhea? If yes, describe your history of this, when it started, how you treated it, etc.

PMS: _____

_____

_____

Other: _____

_____

_____

Do you have weight gains and losses?
PMS: _____

_____

_____

Other: _____

_____

_____

Do you suffer from headaches? If yes, what kind, where, how often, what helps it?
PMS: _____

_____

_____

Other: _____

_____

_____

Do you have any problems with depression? If yes, when, how severe, are you being treated for it, is it all month long or just premenstrually?
PMS: _____

_____

_____

Other: _____

_____

_____

Do you have any problems with anxiety? If yes, when, how severe, are you being treated for it, is it all month long or just premenstrually?
PMS: _____

_____

_____

Other:_____

_____

_____

Do you have crying spells? If yes, when are they most likely to happen, are they "out of nowhere" or are they related to something specific?

PMS: _____

_____

_____

Other:_____

_____

_____

Do you have problems with irritability or with your temper? If yes, when is it most likely to happen? Do you feel badly or guilty after an outburst? Do you feel like a different person while it is happening?

PMS: _____

_____

_____

Other:_____

_____

_____

Do you have any problems with memory and concentration? If yes, does it happen all the time or just at certain times of the month?

PMS: _____

_____

_____

Other:_____

_____

_____

Do you have any lower back problems? If yes, when and how long have you had them?

PMS: _____

_____

_____

Other:_____

_____

_____

Do you have any bone, muscle, or orthopedic problems that prevent you from participating in a regular exercise program?

_____

_____

Do you have frequent vaginal infections? If yes, how many and how often? When are you most likely to get them? When did you get the first infection? How was it treated?

_____

_____

Do you have benign breast disease (lumpy or cystic swellings)?

_____

_____

Do the lumps or cysts change with your cycle?

_____

_____

Do you have cravings at any time of the month? If yes, what kinds and at what point in your cycle?

_____

_____

_____

Is your period irregular in any way? If yes, describe how. When did the irregularity start?

_____

_____

_____

Do you suspect or know that you have allergies? If yes, to what extent and how long have you had them?

_____

_____

_____

Are you aware of sensitivities to pollutants such as car exhaust, gasoline vapors, perfumes, cleaning products, plastics, etc.?

_____

_____

Are there any foods that cause you problems? If yes, what foods and what symptoms do you experience?

_____

_____

_____

Have you taken antibiotics? What kinds? How often? For what kinds of infections?

_____

_____

_____

Have you ever been on the birth control pill? If yes, for how long and when? Were there any problems associated with it? When? Why did you stop taking the pill?

_____

_____

_____

Are you on any medication at the present? What types and for how long?

_____

_____

Have you ever had any unwanted reactions to medication? What happened?

_____

_____

_____

_____

Do you presently take vitamins and nutrients? If yes, what are you taking and have you noticed any difference in how you feel?

_____

_____

Do you exercise regularly? If yes, does it help your PMS symptoms?

_____

_____

Are you willing to start an exercise program?

_____

_____

Do you smoke cigarettes? If yes, how long have you smoked and how many per day?

_____

_____

Do you consume caffeine in the form of coffee, tea, soda, chocolate, etc.? If yes, list how much of each per day.

_____

_____

_____

Do you drink alcohol? If yes, how much, how often, and what kind? Have you had any problems as the result of drinking alcohol?

_____

_____

_____

When was the last time you had a complete physical examination?

_____

_____

When was the last time you had a blood test or urinalysis done?

_____

_____

What were the results of those tests?

_____

_____

_____

_____

Other problems:

_____

_____

_____

_____

PAST PERSONAL HISTORY

Did your mother have any problems when she was pregnant with you or with the delivery?

_____

_____

Describe your general health during childhood. Include common childhood illnesses, frequency of colds, flus, earaches, etc., as well as out of the ordinary illnesses.

_____

_____

_____

_____

Describe your health as an adolescent.

_____

_____

_____

How old were you when you had your first period?

_____

_____

Describe any symptoms associated with menses in the first year or two.

_____

_____

Did these symptoms change over the years? If yes, describe how they changed; lessened, worsened, etc.

_____

_____

_____

_____

Describe your health as an adult.

_____

_____

_____

_____

Have you ever been pregnant?

_____

_____

Have you ever had an abortion? Have you ever had a miscarriage?

_____

_____

Did your PMS symptoms change after the pregnancy? In what way?

_____

_____

What treatments have you tried for your PMS symptoms in the past? What were the results?

_____

_____

_____

Have you ever had any allergy treatment? What kind? Was it helpful?

_____

_____

FAMILY HISTORY

How is your mother's health in general? List any specific problems.

_____

_____

Have any of your female relatives (mother, sisters, aunts, etc.) reported any problems with PMS?

_____

_____

How is your father's health? List any specific problems.

_____

_____

How is the health of your siblings? List any specific problems.

_____

_____

CONCLUSION

Do you feel your main problem is:

☐ PMS
☐ PMS and suspected allergies
☐ PMS and suspected intestinal yeast
☐ Other _____

KEEPING A DIARY

Most women—even those who are certain that they have PMS—have very little sense of how long their periods last, how long their cycles are, when their premenstrual problems in general appear and recede each month, or when each of the different symptoms appears, peaks, and disappears. In other words, they have little idea of their own cycles and symptoms, regardless of how alert they are in other ways.

This is surprising, though it is commonplace. Women are highly skilled at forgetting about their premenstrual problems, either consciously or subconsciously. When the problems are upon us, premenstrual women say, they are all too real and seem, somehow, to *be* our entire lives. But when they are gone, that part of life becomes "other," difficult to remember, difficult to relate to, something that won't happen again.

Women often tell us that as soon as their PMS is over for the month, the experience evaporates completely from their minds. As well, they cannot relate any information about it at all. Not just to us, the professionals; they do not have any information even for themselves. They try to describe what went on during their PMS time, what their problems and symptoms were, but they are woefully—and amazingly—unable to do so. For your doctor to treat you, you must remember what your symptoms are; we suggest that you keep a diary.

We make extensive use of the diary. We recommend it for anyone who thinks she may be premenstrual as it will serve as a tool. It is informative without necessarily being intrusive. From the diary you will learn whether your cycle is regular from month to month, and how long it is. You will learn about your symptoms, how often they occur, how long they last, how intense they are, and eventually what nutrients they respond to best. You will learn, in short, about your own body.

The symptoms you list should include occurrences of acne, anxiety, bloating, breast tenderness, constipation or diarrhea, cramps, crying, depression, changes in energy level, headaches, irritability, changes in sexual interest and responsiveness, lower back pain, nausea or vomiting, and vaginal discharge. When a premenstrual woman first sees this list, there is often an incredible sense of relief; relief because it is now possible to recognize and give a name to the problems she has been dealing with every month.

We suggest that a woman fill in her diary every evening before going to sleep. It is a simple process requiring no more than five minutes. You will find some samples of a diary on the following pages.

The diary has a rating scale that goes from 1 to 10, with 1 as the "best" something gets, and 10 as the "worst." The diary is totally subjective, after all, who can better judge her hunger, tiredness, or irritability than the individual herself?

Up at the top of the diary sheet is a blank space for nutrients. Any nutrients or other medications being taken that week are written in here, then checked off day by day. This is intended as an aid for keeping track of the nutrients being taken, as well as to help determine which nutrients at what dosages have what effects.

On the bottom of each page are other aspects of daily life, such as alcohol consumption, appetite, exercise, cravings, sleep, temperature, weight, birth control pills, and so on.

When the diary pages have been filled out for about three months, it becomes relatively easy to see the patterns that are premenstrual, those that are menstrual, and those that lie completely outside of these cycles. (These are a revelation in themselves.) Typical responses are: "I just never realized I'm irritable the week I thought I was fine," or "I always thought I was terrible for two weeks, but now I see it's more of a gradual build-up and I'm really bad for only five days." The diary clarifies the symptoms, gives a more accurate picture of the cycle, and beyond that, brings things out into the open. The very process of filling out the diary, as well as reviewing the weeks that have gone by to discern the patterns, is an eye-opener. Finally, it makes people aware that as hard as they may try to ignore their PMS times, they are real.

Women who are monitoring themselves should keep a diary roughly similar to those we've illustrated for as long as possible. Our patients usually continue filling out the diaries long after they've left us. Then, if they run into questions or problems, they can call on us or any other physician for help. With the diary as a tool, problem areas can be pinpointed.

There is one other point we want to make about the diaries: Sometimes women decide to use the back of these diary pages for an emotional as well as a physical diary. They find it useful and comforting to correlate their cycles and their emotional life—their fights, their triumphs, and their feelings. Using the diary as both a physical and emotional record-keeping device can sort out which fights, for example, were exaggerated because of premenstrual stress and which ones had nothing to do with body chemistry.

Women who bloat up before their periods are often particularly cheered by the diaries. Sometimes it seems that their weight gain is more than it actually is. They bloat 5 pounds and feel as if they have put on 20. The imagined 20 pounds is terrible for their self-image, resulting in their feeling fat. They keep an extra set of "fat clothes," and they are frustrated. The daily record-keeping helps these women get a grip on how much—or how little—they actually gain. They find out that they are in control. "I'm so fat now," they say, "but at least I'll deflate in a few days." By the fourth month of taking nutrients, the bloating is almost always under control and no longer an issue.

Women should keep a diary for at least one month before starting on a nutrient program. That way they can establish what their "normal" patterns are, find out what has been happening to their bodies "naturally." It is also a way of making sure that they are premenstrual—that their symptoms are cyclical—although most women know whether or not their problems are synchronized with their periods or not. For women who are unwilling to wait a month—and there are many who don't want to wait any longer than they already have—we ask that they recreate a month from memory.

On the following pages there are some completed diary pages to illustrate a typical month of a PMS sufferer. There are some blank diary pages in the appendix.

KEEPING A FOOD DIARY

In addition to our regular PMS diaries, we also ask our patients to keep food diaries. We find it very helpful for them to keep track of what they eat and drink for a period of several weeks. This provides us with important information on which to base dietary suggestions, and can also be helpful in determining if other problems such as food allergies or sensitivities exist.

Food diaries are simple to keep. The diary itself consists of one page that divides each day into five possible eating periods for each day over a seven-day period. The eating periods are:

1.   Morning: This period includes what a person has first thing in the morning, whether it be a big breakfast or just a glass of juice. Also it includes any late morning snacks, whether it be a cup of coffee or a roll with butter. Be sure to include what you put into your coffee or tea if not taken black.

2.   Lunch: This period includes the noon time meal. Some people skip it, while others may make it the largest meal of the day.

PRE-MENSTRUAL SYNDROME – WEEKLY DIARY

Start Date: _April 5_   Finish Date: _April 11_

Day of Cycle	Day 1		Day 2		Day 3		Day 4		Day 5		Day 6		Day 7	
Nutrients:	am	pm	am	pm	am	pm	am	pm	am	pm	am	pm	am	pm
Day of the Week	(Sun.)		(Mon.)		(Tues)		(Wed)		(Thu)		(Fri)		(Sat)	

Indicate Symptom Intensity
(1–10) 1 = Best; 10 = Worst

	am	pm	am	pm	am	pm	am	pm	am	pm	am	pm	am	pm
Acne	7	7	7	6	6	6	6	5	5	5	4	4	4	3
Anxiety	7	7	5	5	4	3	1	1	1	1	1	1	1	1
Bloating	8	8	5	2	1	1	1	1	1	1	1	1	1	1
Breast Tenderness	9	9	6	6	5	4	1	1	1	1	1	1	1	1
Constipation; Diarrhea	0	0	0	0	0	0	0	0	0	0	0	0	0	0
Cramps	10	10	10	8	6	0	0	0	0	0	0	0	0	0
Crying (No. of times)	2	1	0	0	0	0	0	0	0	0	0	0	0	0
Depression	8	5	0	0	0	0	0	0	0	0	0	0	0	0
Energy Level	9	9	9	7	5	5	4	4	4	3	2	2	2	2
Headache	7	7	0	0	0	0	0	0	0	0	0	0	0	0
Irritability; Mood Changes	8	6	4	2	2	1	1	1	1	1	1	1	1	1
Sexual Responsiveness	8	2	2	2	2	2	2	2	2	2	2	2	2	2
Lower Back Pain	7	4	2	2	2	2	2	2	2	2	2	2	2	2
Nausea; Vomiting	5	3	0	0	0	0	0	0	0	0	0	0	0	0
Vaginal Discharge	5	4	0	0	0	0	0	0	0	0	0	0	0	0
Alcohol (# of oz.)		1												
Appetite (1–10)	8	8	7	5	5	5	5	5	5	5	5	5	5	5
Cravings (1–10)	7	7	7	4	3	2	1	1	1	1	1	1	1	1
Exercise (# of min.)							½							½
The Pill (✔)														
Sleep (# of hours)		9		7½		7½		8		8		8		8
Temperature														
Weight	134		133		132		130		130		130		130	
Days of Menstruation (✔)	✔		✔		✔		✔		✔					

PATIENT'S NAME _____

PRE-MENSTRUAL SYNDROME – WEEKLY DIARY

Start Date: _April 12_   Finish Date: _April 18_

Day of Cycle	Day 8		Day 9		Day 10		Day 11		Day 12		Day 13		Day 14	
Nutrients:	am	pm	am	pm	am	pm	am	pm	am	pm	am	pm	am	pm
Day of the Week	(Sun)		(Mon)		(Tue)		(Wed)		(Thu)		(Fri)		(Sat)	

Indicate Symptom Intensity
(1–10) 1 = Best; 10 = Worst

	am	pm	am	pm	am	pm	am	pm	am	pm	am	pm	am	pm
Acne	1	1	1	1	1	1	1	1	1	1	1	1	1	2
Anxiety	1	1	1	1	1	2	1	4	1	1	1	1	3	4
Bloating	1	1	1	1	1	1	1	1	2	2	1	1	2	3
Breast Tenderness	1	1	1	1	1	1	1	1	1	1	1	1	1	1
Constipation; Diarrhea	0	0	0	0	0	0	0	0	0	0	0	0	0	0
Cramps	0	0	0	0	0	0	0	0	0	0	0	0	0	0
Crying (No. of times)	0	0	0	0	0	0	0	0	0	0	0	0	0	0
Depression	3	1	2	1	1	1	1	1	2	1	1	1	2	3
Energy Level	2	2	2	2	2	2	2	2	2	3	3	2	3	4
Headache	0	0	0	0	0	0	0	0	0	0	0	0	0	2
Irritability; Mood Changes	1	1	1	2	2	1	3	1	1	1	2	1	4	4
Sexual Responsiveness	2	2	2	2	2	2	2	2	3	3	2	3	4	4
Lower Back Pain	0	0	0	0	0	0	0	0	0	0	0	0	1	1
Nausea; Vomiting	0	0	0	0	0	0	0	0	0	0	0	0	1	1
Vaginal Discharge	0	0	0	0	0	0	0	0	0	0	0	0	0	0

Alcohol (# of oz.)		1												
Appetite (1–10)	5	5	5	5	5	5	5	5	5	5	5	5	4	4
Cravings (1–10)	0	0	0	1	1	0	0	0	1	1	0	0	0	0
Exercise (# of min.)	1/2						1/2						1/2	
The Pill (✔)														
Sleep (# of hours)		7½		8		7½		8		8		7		7
Temperature														
Weight	130		130		130		130		130		130		130	
Days of Menstruation (✔)														

PATIENT'S NAME _____

PRE-MENSTRUAL SYNDROME – WEEKLY DIARY

Start Date: _April 19_   Finish Date: _April 25_

Day of Cycle	Day 15		Day 16		Day 17		Day 18		Day 19		Day 20		Day 21	
Nutrients:	am	pm	am	pm	am	pm	am	pm	am	pm	am	pm	am	pm
Day of the Week	(Sun)		(Mon)		(Tue)		(Wed)		(Thu)		(Fri)		(Sat)	

Indicate Symptom Intensity
(1–10) 1 = Best; 10 = Worst

	am	pm	am	pm	am	pm	am	pm	am	pm	am	pm	am	pm
Acne	2	2	2	3	1	1	1	1	2	1	1	1	1	1
Anxiety	4	4	4	4	1	1	1	1	2	2	1	1	1	1
Bloating	4	4	4	4	4	4	5	5	5	5	5	4	4	3
Breast Tenderness	3	3	3	2	2	1	1	1	1	1	1	3	3	3
Constipation; Diarrhea	o	o	o	o	o	o	o	o		c		c		c
Cramps	o	o	o	o	o	o	o	o	o	o	o	o	o	o
Crying (No. of times)	o	o	o	o	o	o	o	o	o	o	o	o	o	1
Depression	3	3	2	2	2	1	1	3	3	1	1	4	5	6
Energy Level	4	4	4	4	4	4	4	4	4	5	5	5	5	5
Headache	o	o	o	o	o	o	o	o	o	o	o	o	o	o
Irritability; Mood Changes	4	4	3	4	7	2	2	2	2	2	3	3	2	2
Sexual Responsiveness	4	4	4	3	3	2	2	2	2	2	2	2	2	2
Lower Back Pain	o	o	o	o	o	o	o	o	o	o	o	o	o	o
Nausea; Vomiting	o	o	o	o	o	o	o	o	o	o	o	o	o	o
Vaginal Discharge	o	o	o	o	o	o	o	o	o	o	o	o	1	1

Alcohol (# of oz.)		1												
Appetite (1–10)	5	5	6	6	7	7	6	6	5	5	5	5	5	5
Cravings (1–10)	o	o	3	2	5	5	4	4	2	2	2	1	1	1
Exercise (# of min.)	½							½				½		
The Pill (✓)														
Sleep (# of hours)		8		9		7½		7½		8		8		8
Temperature														
Weight	131		131		131		131		131		131		131	
Days of Menstruation (✓)														

PATIENT'S NAME _____

PRE-MENSTRUAL SYNDROME – WEEKLY DIARY

Start Date: _April 26_   Finish Date: _May 2_

Day of Cycle	Day 22		Day 23		Day 24		Day 25		Day 26		Day 27		Day 28	
Nutrients:	am	pm	am	pm	am	pm	am	pm	am	pm	am	pm	am	pm
Day of the Week	(Sun)		(Mon)		(Tue)		(Wed)		(Thu)		(Fri)		(Sat)	

Indicate Symptom Intensity
(1–10) 1 = Best; 10 = Worst

	am	pm	am	pm	am	pm	am	pm	am	pm	am	pm	am	pm
Acne	1	1	2	2	3	4	4	4	5	5	5	5	6	6
Anxiety	1	1	1	2	4	5	5	5	7	7	7	7	7	7
Bloating	3	3	4	4	5	5	7	7	8	8	8	8	8	8
Breast Tenderness	3	3	4	4	5	5	7	7	8	8	8	8	8	8
Constipation; Diarrhea	o	o	o	o	o	o	o	c	c	c	c	c	c	D
Cramps	o	o	o	o	o	o	o	o	o	o	o	4	4	4
Crying (No. of times)	o	o	o	1	o	o	o	1	1	1	o	1	o	1
Depression	6	6	7	7	7	7	8	8	8	8	8	8	8	8
Energy Level	5	5	6	6	7	7	8	8	9	9	9	9	9	9
Headache	o	o	o	1	2	1	o	o	o	3	0	7	o	o
Irritability; Mood Changes	2	2	3	4	7	8	8	8	8	8	8	8	8	8
Sexual Responsiveness	2	2	2	5	7	7	7	7	7	7	7	5	5	5
Lower Back Pain	o	o	o	o	o	4	4	4	4	4	4	4	4	4
Nausea; Vomiting	o	o	o	o	o	o	o	o	o	o	2	2	3	3
Vaginal Discharge	o	o	o	o	o	o	o	4	4	4	4	4	4	4
Alcohol (# of oz.)		1				2				2				
Appetite (1–10)	5	5	7	7	8	8	9	10	10	10	10	10	10	10
Cravings (1–10)	3	3	4	4	4	5	7	7	7	7	7	7	7	7
Exercise (# of min.)		1/2												
The Pill (✓)														
Sleep (# of hours)		9		9		10		9		9		8 1/2		9
Temperature														
Weight	132		132		133		134		134		134		134	
Days of Menstruation (✓)														

PATIENT'S NAME _____

3. Afternoon: This period includes anything eaten between the noon and evening meals. Include all snacks and beverages.

4. Dinner: This is the evening meal, and for many people the most substantial of the day.

5. Evening snack: The evening snack includes whatever a person eats from dinner until bedtime. This is when one usually consumes the ice cream and cookies. Of course, anything eaten after dinner until morning should be included here—in case you eat in the middle of the night.

The important thing is for you to record *all* foods or beverages consumed in a 24-hour period.

We have found that tracking your diet serves a very real purpose. Many people really have no idea of what and how much they eat in a day. Often, keeping a food diary (even for just a few weeks) forces you to see and remember what and how much you are consuming. As a result, you are able to make decisions about your diet using the information available to you. We suggest you make changes after you see what you have been eating for several weeks.

Our suggestion for anyone who suspects they suffer from PMS is to keep an account of your diet while on the nutritional program. For the person suffering from PMS, the diet diary will help you notice when you have cravings and for which specific foods and beverages.

Food diaries are helpful in understanding your eating patterns and will give you a greater awareness and more control over your eating and drinking habits.

**SELF-
EVALUATION**

If you are thinking about self-treatment for PMS, we advise you to see your doctor first. Tell him or her about your symptoms and why you think they indicate premenstrual syndrome. Show your doctor your physical diary, or a chart of your symptoms. If he or she is not familiar with PMS, refer him or her to this book or to our suggested readings or references (listed in the appendix).

Tell your doctor about the nutrient program and ask if he or she will oversee you during it. Get a partnership going. You will find that most doctors appreciate a knowledgeable, interested patient who takes some of the responsibility for her own health. Enlist the doctor's help and ask if he or she will do a series of lab tests to ascertain whether you have underlying problems. Thyroid malfunction, hidden infection, and anemia are the main things to look for. These tests will also show whether you have certain vitamin deficiencies. Ask your doctor to consider the following tests:

- a pap test
- a thyroid screen
- a complete blood count
- a chem-screen profile (a blood test that measures minerals, cholesterol, proteins, sugars, etc.)
- a urinalysis

You should also have your height, weight, and blood pressure on record.

**FINDING A
DOCTOR**

In most cases, your family doctor can be the person to oversee you in this program. If you suspect you have an intestinal yeast problem or allergies, then we recommend you find a specialist who is familiar with these and is trained to deal with them. In our experience, the best-trained physicians for dealing with allergies are environmental medicine specialists. If you need help locating one near you, we have provided the address of the American Academy of Environmental Medicine in the appendix. They can provide you with the names of physicians in your area (U.S. and Canada).

If your family doctor is unwilling or unable to work with you on this program, then you may want to seek out someone who will. Finding a physician who you can work with and trust is important, and is worth every effort put into it. The following section deals with how to find a physician. The information presented is important in finding both a general physician as well as a specialist.

What You're Looking For

The way people go about finding a physician today differs drastically from the ways used a hundred years ago. In the past, people went to the only doctor in town, or the one who treated their parents, or relatives, or to one recommended by a friend.

Today, medicine is greatly dependent on specialists, and general or family practitioners can be very hard to find. Huge amounts of new information have had to be incorporated into medical practice and specialization has provided the means for doing this. Unfortunately, consumers frequently don't understand the resulting cubbyholes and don't know where to look for the doctor who can help them. They trek from one specialist to another, looking for answers, with a growing sense of frustration and a pile of bills.

Specialists sometimes cannot, or else choose not to coordinate the different types of care that are needed. Some physicians explain carefully what they are planning or what they have done. We're hopeful that a new trend towards making these connections is developing, and that the practice of family medicine will be redefined and revitalized by physicians who think the relationship between you and your primary doctor is crucial.

You need a general physician who will treat you for most problems and will know when to refer you to a specialist (and which one), and who will act as your advocate throughout the medical system. You should look for a good internist or family or general practitioner. He or she will help you find integrated health care rather than scattered attention, with its possible duplication, missed problems, and high costs that are a burden either to you or to the medicare system.

How To Find the Right Doctor

The search for a physican represents an investment in your health. You should research and compare choices just as you would if you were buying a house. Do not settle for a physician you know nothing about. Your decision can have valuable results for your health. Start by asking your friends and neighbors about their physicians. Some of your questions should concern:

1. training and background
2. whether other patients have been satisfied with their care
3. personality and style
4. costs (if you are not covered by a health plan or medicare)

Did other patients feel rushed? Listened to? Comfortable enough to be fully honest about what ailed them? Keep in mind that your neighbor may prefer a doctor who resembles his great-uncle, and your cousin may want someone she can talk philosophy with in the examining room. Gather as many impressions as you can.

Call the best hospitals near you, or the hospital to which you would choose to go, if necessary. Ask for a list of internists and family practitioners who have hospital privileges. Medical centers may offer higher quality care, in an atmosphere of learning and discovery.

Community hospitals may provide more personal attention. Each may be appropriate for different needs.

Get lists of names. Check the doctors out with the local medical society, hospitals, and public interest groups. If you're certain you need a specialist, find out who the doctors' families see for a particular problem. Nurses are often a knowledgeable resource about the physicians in their area.

Assessing the Possibilities

You can save time initially by calling several doctors' offices and talking with their secretaries or receptionists. First, ask if the person you've reached is busy; if so, ask whether you could call back when they have some time to answer your questions. Formulate some general questions that will help you determine what a suitable doctor for you is. Ask the person at the other end of the phone if the doctor offers the type of care you want. A secretary may reflect her employer's attitude and interests. If the person who answers the phone sounds rude, uninterested or unwilling to talk with you, that may give you important information about the doctor. On the other hand, someone who can answer your questions courteously will help you decide whether to investigate the office further.

The most important step in making a decision is arranging a talk with the physician in person. Tell the receptionist that you have some questions and would like to see the doctor when he or she isn't rushed. If the doctor is too busy to see you, even for a nominal office visit fee, then he or she may be too busy for your needs. Often, young physicians, just starting a practice will have time to develop the right kind of relationship.

You're probably not looking for someone who only gives directions; you want a partner. Pay attention to your own personality, as well as that of the doctor, and to the way you affect each other. Are you the type of person who forgets all of your questions when you reach the office and who needs to make several phone calls later? Does the physician, or the secretary mind this habit? Do you need to be offered several treatment alternatives, with their advantages and drawbacks, and then come to your own decision? Or would you rather have your physician make the final choices? Have you felt uncomfortable or reluctant in describing certain physical symptoms? Does this doctor help you express yourself?

Be prepared when you go to the physician's office, whether for an interview or for an examination. Write down questions, or symptoms you want to talk about. Take notes. Have a good sense of what you want to communicate so you can help the doctor do a good job on your behalf. Your "performance" as a patient needs to be organized and prepared, in the same way that you want the physician to be organized and prepared for his or her part.

We are outlining many of the factors that you should consider in making your choice of a physician. As with any endeavor, you will have to decide which factors are musts and which ones are desirable, but not crucial. You may even want to use a rating scale as you consider each physician.

1. How well were you treated by the doctor's staff?
2. How well organized are the office and personnel?
3. Was there a rushed feeling?
4. Does the doctor run behind schedule?
5. Did you mind waiting?
6. What was your first impression of the doctor?
7. Did you feel more or less relaxed than what is usual for you in a physician's office?
8. Could you talk with reasonable ease?
9. Is the doctor a good listener?
10. How thorough does he/she seem?

11. What was your impression of his/her organization?
12. Did you get an explanation (one you could understand) of the diagnosis or treatment plans?
13. Overall, how did the visit go, and how did you feel about it?

All of these questions are important in deciding on the right physician for you. It is important to remember that the perfect doctor does not exist. What you are looking for is a good doctor who takes the time to give you all the information you need and the time for both of you to make intelligent decisions about your health.

SPECIAL PROBLEMS ASSOCIATED WITH PMS

As we have mentioned throughout this book, PMS can present special problems in the relationship between you and your doctor. Not all doctors believe that PMS exists, and many will try to dismiss it or steer you in a different direction. It is sometimes hard to distinguish between a statement that is based on good medical sense and one that is based on rejecting PMS as a medical problem. The best way to find out is to ask your doctor directly what his or her feelings are about PMS. Does he/she view it as a medical condition that can be treated? Is he or she knowledgeable about it? Is he or she interested in learning more about it? If the answer to these questions is yes, and the doctor still feels that your condition represents another medical problem, then we suggest you follow through on his or her suggestion, and rule out the other condition before going to a PMS diagnosis.

If your physician tells you outright that there is no such thing as PMS and that it's just the price you pay for being a woman, find another doctor.

If your problem is complicated by either a suspected intestinal yeast condition or environmental allergies, you will probably need to find an environmental specialist familiar with these conditions to get the proper treatment. As mentioned earlier in this section, we have provided the names, addresses, and phone numbers for the American Academy of Environmental Medicine in the appendix. When you get a list of names, be sure to apply the same criteria and questions we have discussed here in selecting the right doctor.

Environmental medicine specialists often have expertise in treating PMS from a nutritional perspective. If you are unable to locate a family practitioner who is willing to oversee such a program, you may want to consider an environmental medicine specialist to work with on nutritional treatment as well.

In our practice, we offer (at no charge) information sessions with a staff member for prospective patients. This serves several important purposes. First, it allows the prospective patient the time to get to know us and to gain an understanding of what we do and how we do it. It's a time to have questions answered, and it affords the patient a chance of getting a sense of who we are, what our style is like, and if they feel comfortable with us. It provides patients with the opportunity to discover first hand whether this is the place for them to have their problem treated.

The information session also gives us the opportunity to assess whether or not our office is the place where this patient ought to be. It may be obvious that there is a problem that should be treated by a different specialist and these sessions allow us to make that suggestion to the patient before she has spent any time or money. With rising health-care costs, this kind of free information session is beneficial to most patients.

ONE STEP AT A TIME   One of our problems as medical consumers is that we've gotten used to taking recommended dosages of medicines, be they drugs, nutrients, or vitamins. We assume that the recommended dosage just happens to be the best one for our individual needs. But taking a recommended dosage is not necessarily the right dosage; most of the time, it is not the *optimal* dosage for *any* individual.

One of the cornerstones of our approach is that optimal relief is the goal of treatment. Therefore, we want our patients to take nutrients at dosages that are optimal for their individual metabolism and needs. For everyone to take the same dosage is comparable to everyone trying to fit into the same size shoes, slacks or dress.

The method we use to find an individual's optimal dosage is a graduated approach. It simply involves beginning with a very low dosage of a substance and gradually increasing it until the system reacts. Then the dosage is lowered slightly.

One of the great values of this approach is that it pinpoints precisely what *your* body needs, not what someone else's body needs. The amount of primrose oil that you need, for instance, may be considerably different from the dosage your neighbor needs. To say that everyone should take three primrose oil capsules a day would be cheating people out of the best possible treatment. It would help a few people, but it would not be the optimal dosage for many.

What the graduated approach offers is optimal amounts of nutrients for your system. It enables you to determine what you actually need. Each of us can learn to be observant of our own bodies and the changes we go through, and of the effects of various foods, drugs, nutrients and activities. The graduated approach can and should be used with as many of the nutrients as possible.

Beyond that, we always have our patients split up their vitamin dosages. Vitamins are taken twice a day, half the dosage at a time instead of all at once. Splitting the dosage is especially important for the water-soluble nutrients like vitamin C and the B vitamins. We advise people to take these vitamins two or three times throughout the day rather than all at once.

Most people take vitamins in the morning and think they've taken their vitamins for the day. But what they are not taking into account is that three or four hours after they've swallowed the pills, half of the substance has already been eliminated from their system. As for pills that are time-released, you may as well be eating candy, some nutritionists say, as the timing is all too often inadequate. (The pills can sometimes be seen intact in the bowel movement later on that day.)

Finally, vitamins should not be taken on an empty stomach; a negative reaction to vitamins is frequently the result. We suggest you eat something first and then take the vitamins.

THE ALL IMPORTANT CO-FACTORS

Co-factors are nutrients that work together to make something happen. In the case of PMS, it is the conversion of essential fatty acids to prostaglandin E-1 that requires certain co-factors. Co-factors necessary for this conversion are vitamin C (which is needed during the conversion of linoleic acid to gammalinolenic acid), vitamin B_6 (pyridoxine), vitamin B_3 (niacin), and zinc.

Vitamin C

We start everyone with 500 to 3000 milligrams (mg) of vitamin C per day, depending mostly on whether they smoke, and/or drink, and on the kinds of stress they are under. Both tobacco and alcohol deplete the store of vitamin C rapidly, so if a woman smokes and/or drinks, we generally recommend a considerably higher dosage of this vitamin than if she does not. In addition, because vitamin C is water soluble and does not remain in the system for a long period of time, we use a split dosage, with half to be taken in the morning and the other half at night. Vitamin C offers a fringe benefit, as we firmly believe it increases the body's defenses against influenza, colds, and other upper-respiratory ailments.

If a patient smokes cigarettes or drinks more than two ounces of alcohol a day (that's the equivalent of about one mixed drink, or two beers, or two glasses of wine), we recommend that the dosage be gradually built up to 3000 mg of vitamin C per day. Otherwise, we usually stop at 2000 mg daily. Sensitivity to vitamin C generally shows up as stomach discomfort, gaseousness, or diarrhea. Usually, it is only megadoses, in the range of 8000 to 10,000 mg daily, that bring on these symptoms, although some people do not tolerate more than 500 mg per day. Symptoms of vitamin C sensitivity are, of course, an indication that the dosage should be lowered. Do not take over 4000 mg of vitamin C per day.

The B Vitamins

The B vitamins, sometimes known as the "energy vitamins," are of special importance to women who tend to feel lethargic and tired, sometimes premenstrually, sometimes without apparent connection to their menstrual cycle. For vegetarian women, supplements of the B vitamins may be particularly important because one of them, B_{12}, is extremely difficult to obtain from any source other than meat.

There are eight different B vitamins; they must be present in a particular ratio to work most efficiently. (See the following chart for sample ratios. Not all B complexes will be exactly in these ratios, but they should be similar.) Vitamin B-complex pills should contain all of the B vitamins in appropriate ratios. We have found that trying to take each of the B vitamins separately is usually problematic. Unfortunately, the balance is easily thrown off by even the most careful practitioner, and it is not unusual to find someone taking far too much of some of the Bs and not enough of the others. We recommend beginning with a 50-Balance B-complex vitamin based on 50 mg of thiamine and riboflavin; the rest are matched proportionately to that base figure. Usually we recommend an upper limit of two 50-Balance B-complexes daily.

Typical 50-Balance Vitamin B-Complex Ratios
B_1 (Thiamine): 50 mg
B_2 (Riboflavin): 50 mg
B_3 (Niacin, Nicotinic acid, Nicotinamide): 150 mg
B_6 (Pyridoxine, Pyridoxal, Pyridoxamine): 100 mg
B_{12} (Cobalamin, Cyanocobalamin): 200 mg
Folic acid (Folacin, Folate): 400 mcg
Biotin: 200 mcg
Pantothenic acid: 100 mg

Vitamin B_6

There is one B vitamin that we recommend taking in addition to the B-complex. This is vitamin B_6, also called pyridoxine. Among other functions, vitamin B_6 has a dampening effect on prolactin, a hormone associated with the bloating aspects of PMS as well as with breast tenderness or soreness. Prolactin is produced near the time of ovulation, usually on or about Day 15 of the cycle.

Some of the functions of vitamin B_6, according to the *Medical Reference Library, Nutrition and Vitamins*, are the manufacture of proteins from amino acids, the manufacture of "fats" from fatty acids, the formation and functioning of red blood cells, bile salts, over sixty enzymes, and many hormones. Futhermore, B_6 is a co-enzyme in muscle, lymph, liver, and nerve tissue. It also helps maintain the chemical balance in the tissues and the excretion of water (a lack of which causes bloating). It is necessary for the health of bones and skeletal tissue. A deficiency of B6 is said to produce sores of the skin, lips, and tongue, and to produce nervous system disorders, including confusion, nervousness, and depression. The recommended daily allowance (RDA) for vitamin B6 is 2 mg, higher for lactating or pregnant women. Usually, toxicity occurs only after doses as high as one gram per pound of body weight daily. Recent studies, however, have shown that occasionally there may be problems with B6 at dosages of over 250 mg per day.

We start people with 50 mg of vitamin B6 per day, in addition to the vitamin B-complex pills. If bloating is a problem for an individual, we usually recommend an additional 100 mg per day, starting one week before bloating symptoms would normally begin. We do not recommend dosages of over 250 mg per day, except under the careful direction of a physician.

Zinc

Ten milligrams per day of the trace element zinc is another part of our nutrient therapy for PMS. This dosage remains the same for the first full month of treatment, and is then increased to 20 mg per day for the second month, if there have been no adverse reactions. Zinc is then taken in a split dosage, with 10 mg in the morning and another 10 mg at night. It is of particular benefit to women who have acne associated with their PMS.

Sometimes women who have never taken zinc supplements before find it causes slight nausea. This can usually be traced to their taking the zinc on an empty stomach. None of the vitamins should be taken on an empty stomach, but zinc, in particular, can cause symptoms of nausea.

**Evening
Primrose Oil**

PMS could be described most simply as a prostaglandin E-1 problem. Therefore, we use a nutritional supplement that supplies gammalinolenic acid, a precursor of prostaglandin E-1. The most readily available source of gammalinolenic acid (GLA) is the evening primrose (*Oenothera biennis*). Providing GLA directly, in the form of evening primrose oil (made from the seed of the plant), bypasses the body's need to convert linoleic acid from the diet to gammalinolenic acid.

The only other source of gammalinolenic acid in substantial quantities is human breast milk. Two pints (about one liter) of human milk contain only about as much gammalinolenic acid as three capsules of evening primrose oil. Obviously, breast milk is not very practical as a source of gammalinolenic acid. It is intriguing to note, however, its presence in breast milk, and presumably, its value for infant nutritional needs. A woman who is breastfeeding loses large amounts of GLA and closely related fatty acids in her milk. It is possible that this could be one of the factors making PMS worse with successive pregnancies.

Several other oils contain linoleic acid in the form necessary for conversion to gammalinolenic acid, called the *cis* form. Safflower oil contains 73% cis-linoleic acid; corn oil has 57% cis-linoleic acid; and sunflower oil has 58%. For a small percentage of people, these oils—especially safflower oil—in their purest form can be beneficial and therapeutic for the treament of PMS problems. However, the processing of the oils converts some of the fatty acids into a different and unusable form, called the *trans* form. The trans form cannot be converted to gammalinolenic acid (and after that, to prostaglandin E-1). Processed oils, including margarines, block gammalinolenic acid formation and actually interfere with the conversion process.

THE BASIC PROGRAM

For clear-cut cases of PMS, we usually start off with one evening primrose capsule per day. After one week we raise the dosage to two capsules per day. When one starts to correct an essential fatty acid deficiency by taking evening primrose oil, an occasional woman may experience a temporary feeling of lethargy and headache. A *short* period of lethargy and headache, one that lasts for about 24 hours, is not necessarily an indication of a problem, neither is it reason enough to lower the dosage. Few people experience this, however.

Think of the body as being in such need of GLA that when it does get some, it overreacts for a short period of time. Therefore, if a woman experiences headache and lethargy for 24 hours after beginning to take the primrose oil, we generally recommend she continue on the program.

The basic program we recommend for treatment of premenstrual syndrome can be seen below.

| Nutrient & Amount | Day of Cycle | | | |
	1–3	4–11	12–19	20–28
Primrose oil	0	1	2	3
B-Complex 50 or Super Balance	1 a.m.	1 a.m.	1 a.m.	1 a.m.
B₆, 50 mg	0	0	2	2
Zinc, 10 mg	1 a.m.	1 a.m.	1 a.m.	1 a.m.
Vitamin C	500 mg a.m./p.m.	500 mg a.m./p.m.	1000 mg a.m./p.m.	1000 mg a.m./p.m.

If one has difficulty in swallowing capsules (and many people do), a capsule may be broken open and the oil rubbed into the skin. Evening primrose oil is absorbed extremely efficiently through the skin. Rub the oil into the soft skin of the inside arm or the abdomen for fast absorption.

During the first month of the nutrient program, an increase in primrose oil to two or three capsules a day is usually recommended, with the dosage divided into one or two capsules in the morning and one or two at night. Usually, we recommend one in the morning and two at night.

If, after one month, there is some relief from the PMS symptoms, we increase the dosage to four or five capsules a day. Generally, we increase the dosage until we find an individual's tolerance level and then decrease it to just below that level.

The tolerance level is that level above which symptoms of minor side effects appear. As soon as there are side effects, the dosage should be decreased. Side effects from evening primrose oil are very rare, but may include a slight increase in headaches and an occasional feeling of lethargy. (Interestingly enough, during the clinical trials with evening primrose oil and PMS, these side effects were reported equally as often by women taking placebo capsules as by women taking evening primrose oil capsules.) So don't worry if you experience these effects, just lower the dosage slightly. Once established, this tolerance level is used only for the week just prior to menstruation. For the rest of the month, a lower dosage is more appropriate.

Primrose oil is always taken on a gradually building schedule during the month, from Day 4 until Day 1, when it is discontinued for several days. The hormones build up from Day 1 (the beginning of estrogen production) to Day 28. On Days 1 through 4, the lowest amounts of hormones are being produced.

Start the primrose oil on Day 4 or Day 5, then increase it gradually until the final day of the cycle. On Day 1, it should be discontinued entirely, to be resumed on Day 4 or 5. Primrose oil dosage works on a monthly cycle with a two- or three-day period when it is not taken.

The following are typical dosages of primrose oil for clear-cut cases of PMS (cases with no underlying problems):

THE FIRST MONTH

One capsule of primrose oil on Day 4 or Day 5 of the cycle, going on to two capsule per day on Day 12. This is flexible and can be a day earlier or a day later. On Day 20, increase the dosage to three capsules. Continue at three capsules a day until menstruation begins, at which time the primrose oil is discontinued completely until Day 4 or 5.

THE SECOND MONTH

Assuming there has been some success (even though it may be slight at first), the second month begins with one capsule a day on Day 4 or 5. On Day 10, this is increased to two capsules a day. Increase the dosage again on Day 17 or 18 to three capsules a day. On Day 21 or 22, this is raised to four a day. Again, the primrose oil is discontinued on the first day of menstruation (Day 1 of the cycle).

THE THIRD MONTH

If the patient is finding more relief now than during the first month of treatment, then the dosage should be increased slightly. The third month begins with one capsule a day on Day 4 or 5, two beginning on Day 10, three beginning on Day 15 or 16, then four capsules per day beginning on Day 20, and five beginning on Day 23.

This kind of gradual build-up can be continued over a period of several months until the optimum dosage is reached. Always assuming, of course, that more and more relief is being derived from the treatment. Remember, the moment there are side effects, the dosage is decreased.

CO-FACTORS TO USE WITH EPO

The basis of the nutrient program is evening primrose oil, vitamin C, the B vitamins (with special emphasis on B_6), and zinc. However, additional nutrients are sometimes called for. The following chart will illustrate what nutrients can be added based on specific symptoms. This will be followed by a summary of each co-factor nutrient.

Especially if irritability is a component of a woman's PMS, we recommend 500 mg of magnesium per day, to be taken in the morning. Many women choose to buy magnesium in the form of a calcium-magnesium supplement.

SYMPTOM	NUTRIENT AND DOSAGE
Bloating	B_6, 50 mg. Increase to a maximum of 100 mg in the morning and 100 mg at night.
Breast tenderness	Same as for bloating.
Cravings	Chromium, 200–400 mcg. One capsule in the morning and one at night.
Anxiety/Irritability	Magnesium, 500 mg in the morning.
Cramps	Aspirin, one-half tablet each day from Day 10 on.
Insomnia/ Depression	Tryptophan, 500–1500 mg. One at night, to a maximum of 4.

SAMPLE OF BEGINNING NUTRIENT PROGRAM OF EVENING PRIMROSE OIL

Day	1st Month				2nd Month					3rd Month					
	0	1	2	3	0	1	2	3	4	0	1	2	3	4	5
1	x				x					x					
2	x				x					x					
3	x				x					x					
4		x				x					x				
5		x				x					x				
6		x				x					x				
7		x				x					x				
8		x				x					x				
9		x				x					x				
10		x				x					x				
11		x					x					x			
12			x				x					x			
13			x				x					x			
14			x				x						x		
15			x				x						x		
16			x				x						x		
17			x					x					x		
18			x					x					x		
19			x					x					x		
20				x				x						x	
21				x					x					x	
22				x					x					x	
23				x					x						x
24				x					x						x
25				x					x						x
26				x					x						x
27				x					x						x
28				x					x						x
1	x				x					x					
2	x				x					x					
3	x				x					x					

Magnesium

In addition, magnesium is important in the manufacture of proteins and DNA for the production and transfer of energy, for muscle contractions, for normal nerve functions, for building bones and teeth, as a co-factor in the production of enzymes and prostaglandins, and as an aid to the body in adjusting to cold temperatures. It helps keep blood levels of cholesterol low and protects against atherosclerosis. Magnesium is thought to be a preventive of cardiovascular disease, and it also helps to keep blood pressure low. This nutrient is also required for glucose metabolism, and is frequently used in intravenous solutions. Magnesium is a cathartic and dulls the appetite.

Magnesium is found naturally in whole-grain products, nuts, seeds, green, leafy vegetables, and seafood. However, processing, the use of water-softening agents, and heat all remove magnesium. We do not recommend magnesium in the form of dolomite or bone meal because it may contain heavy metal and other environmental contaminants.

Chromium GTF Glucose Intolerance Factor

Useful for those women who experience food cravings, typically for sugars (such as chocolate) and carbohydrates (such as pizza), is supplemental chromium GTF. This trace element is intimately involved in blood-glucose regulation. Although the exact chemical structure of chromium GTF is still being researched, it is known that this glucose tolerance factor is related to diabetes, hypoglycemia, and other blood-glucose problems. According to *Mental and Elemental Nutrients*, a physicians' guide to nutrition by Carl Pfeiffer (1975): ''Many women in Western countries are so deficient in chromium that the white blood cell chromium level may decrease by 50 percent with each pregnancy, resulting first in complete alcohol intolerance and later in glucose intolerance (adult-type diabetes).'' The best sources of chromium GTF are brewer's yeast and sugar-beet molasses.

Vitamin E

Vitamin E is an anti-oxidant, which blocks certain types of oxygen damage to key body constituents, notably fats. It reduces the production of potentially harmful substances known as leukotrienes—unwanted products of essential fatty acid chemistry. The body's requirements for vitamin E are increased if essential fatty acid intake is high, and if supplementary iron is being taken. Vitamin E is present in substantial amounts in evening primrose oil and a further 13.6 IU are added to each capsule just to make sure.

Vitamin E's wide distribution in foods includes vegetable oils, wheat germ, eggs, butter, cereals and broccoli, as well as small amounts in meats, fruits, and other vegetables.

We predict that vitamin E will gain importance in the treatment of benign breast disease. (It has been found that reducing caffeine intake and taking vitamin E can reduce the size of cysts in benign breast disease.) In addition, evidence is accumulating that vitamin E applied locally promotes healing. Many believe that vitamin E is of value in diseases of the heart and circulatory system, as well as in arthritis.

The United States' RDA (recommended daily allowance) for vitamin E is 30 IU per day. Unlike the other fat-soluble vitamins, there is no evidence that even very high doses of vitamin E are toxic, but we recommend that less that 400 IUs of vitamin E be ingested per day.

Tryptophan

When insomnia is part of a PMS problem, we often recommend 500 mg of tryptophan. This dosage must be experimented with, however. Most women find they can handle a high dosage very well. We generally recommend between 500 and 2000 mg, to be taken one hour before bedtime.

Tryptophan is an amino acid, a group of substances from which all proteins are made, and must be used with caution. If a woman finds she has headaches or any other problems that seem to be associated with taking tryptophan, it should be discontinued *immediately*. (To determine if a nutrient is causing the problems, discontinue taking it for two days to see if the symptoms it may be causing disappear. If the problems clear up, then the substance may well be the cause.) Tryptophan is a precursor of serotonin, a neurotransmitter of the brain, elevated levels of which induce drowsiness. There is also evidence that an elevated level of serotonin has an anti-depressant effect.

Aspirin

If premenstrual or menstrual cramping is a problem, we usually recommend half an aspirin per day, beginning on Day 6 or 7 of the cycle and continuing until the middle of the menstrual flow. Aspirin is an effective anti-prostaglandin (or prostaglandin inhibitor) that works on the F series of prostaglandins—those most associated with uterine contractions.

Aspirin is not effective for severe cramps, however, unless it is begun well in advance of the onset of cramps. Women who take as many as eight aspirins per day for menstrual cramps, but only on the days when they are in pain, are unable to get the relief they would derive from just half an aspirin daily taken over a three-week period.

Other anti-prostaglandins that are available over-the-counter are Advil and Nuprin, both of which can be taken with the onset of cramps, following the directions on the labels.

MORE ON THE DIET

Caffeine

In addition, caffeine and other caffeine-containing substances (xanthines) such as chocolate, tea, and many soft drinks, appear to have a significantly negative effect

THE CAFFEINE
CONTENT . . .[6]

In Popular Foods
and Beverages

Item	Milligrams Caffeine
Coffee (5-ounce cup)	
Drip method	110–150
Percolated	64–24
Instant	40–106
Decaffeinated	2–5
Instant Decaffeinated	2
Tea (loose or bags, 5-ounce cup)	
1-minute brew	9–33
3-minute brew	20–46
5-minute brew	20–50
Tea products	
Instant tea (5-ounce cup)	12–28
Iced tea (12-ounce can)	22–36
Cocoa	
Made from mix	6
Milk chocolate (1 ounce)	6
Baking chocolate (1 ounce)	35

In Soft Drinks

Soft Drinks with caffeine	Mg caffeine (per 12-ounce serving)
Sugar-Free Mr. PIBB	58.8
Mountain Dew	54.0
Mello Yello	52.8
TAB	46.8
Coca-Cola	45.6
Diet Coke	45.6
Shasta Cola	44.4
Shasta Cherry Cola	44.4
Shasta Diet Cola	44.4
Shasta Diet Cherry Soda	44.4
Mr. PIBB	40.8
Dr. Pepper	39.6
Sugar-Free Dr. Pepper	39.6
Big Red	38.4
Sugar-Free Big Red	38.4

Pepsi-Cola	38.4
Aspen	36.0
Diet Pepsi	36.0
Pepsi Light	36.0
RC Cola	36.0
Diet Rite	36.0
Kick	31.2
Canada Dry Jamacia Cola	30.0
Canada Dry Diet Cola	1.2

In Drugs

Classification	Mg per tablet or capusule
Stimulants	
NoDoz Tablets	100
Vivarin Tablets	200
Pain Relievers	
Anacin	32
Excedrin	65
Midol	32
Plain aspirin, any brand	0
Vanguish	33
Diuretic	
Aqua-Ban	100
Cold Remedies	
Ceryban-D	30
Dristan	16.2
Triaminicin	30
Weight-control aids	
Dexatrim	200
Dietac	200
Prolamine	140

on premenstrual syndrome. They should probably be avoided. This class of substances cause muscle tissues to contract and elicits a merry-go-round of short bursts of energy followed by periods of tiredness and tightness. The person who ingests caffeine often ends up feeling "uptight" and needing another "hit" of coffee, tea, or chocolate.

Some doctors who are researching premenstrual syndrome recommend complete abstinence from the xanthines. In her book, *No More Menstrual Cramps and Other Good News*, Dr. Penny Wise Budoff also advises that the caffeine should be completely avoided. Women should limit their intake of even decaffeinated coffee, because some of these substances are not removed during the decaffeination process. (In addition, recent research has shown that the chemicals used to decaffeinate coffee may be carcinogenic.)

Margarine

Margarine should be avoided. During World War II, butter was in short supply and was partially replaced in our kitchens by margarine. It was solid white and came with a packet of dye that had to be mixed in by the customer.

Margarine is made from a liquid oil that is changed into a firm substance that looks and acts like butter. This process is called *hydrogenation*; it is a method of putting hydrogen into the oil. Hydrogenation, however, renders the oil unusable by the body as a polyunsaturate. At the same time that it is rendered unusable, the hydrogenated oil is competing with the ''good'' oils or fats from elsewhere in the diet. If you ate some margarine that was made of half useless and half usable, health-producing oil, your body would only be able to derive benefit from a small part of the health-producing oil because of interference from the hydrogenated oil. In addition, the effects of the dyes used in margarine may interfere with good health.

The diet followed by sufferers of hypoglycemia (a condition where the body produces too much insulin and over-processed sugars) is often helpful in the treatment of PMS. This diet includes restricted sugar intake, eating frequent small meals and snacks rather than one or two big meals every day, and stresses high carbohydrates, fiber, starches, protein and low-fat foods.

There is also controversy as to what food groups to emphasize. According to some authorities, the diet should be high in starchy carbohydrates and fiber.

POSSIBLE PROBLEMS

Most side effects from these nutrients are a result of either nutrient intolerance or of the nutrients being introduced too quickly. We recommend very low dosages that are gradually built up over a period of several months. We found that this method is much more comfortable for most people. It also enables us to gain greater awareness and control over our bodies. In fact, it is important that we learn to be observant about how each nutrient, at each dosage, is affecting us.

The single greatest source of side effects from the nutrients is from having taken them on an empty stomach. *We cannot stress enough that many individuals should not ingest nutrients until after a substantial breakfast—or at least something of some substance —has been eaten.* In the evening this is not crucial as there is some food in the system from earlier in the day. Some people are, of course, able to take them at any time without any difficulty.

Certain medications can interfere with the effects of the vitamins we take, and vice versa, so it is important to consult a doctor if you are considering taking vitamins and other medication. Below is a partial list of known drug/vitamin interactions.

DRUGS AND OTHER SUBSTANCES	VITAMINS THEY INTERACT WITH[7]
Antacids	Vitamin C
Antibiotics	Most B vitamins, vitamin K
Anticoagulants	Vitamin C, vitamin K, vitamin E
Anticonvulsants	Vitamin D

Antidepressants	Vitamin C
Anti-diabetic agents (oral)	Vitamin C can increase their effects
Aspirin, aspirin substitutes	Vitamins K, B12, C
Baking soda	Vitamin B1
Chloramphenicol	Vitamin B12
Codeine	Vitamin B12
Contraceptives (oral)	Vitamins C, E, B1, B2, B6, B12, and folic acid
Cortisone and Prednisone	Vitamins C, B6, and D
Diuretics	Vitamin C
Hydralazine	Vitamin B6
Indomethacin	Vitamin C
Iron	Vitamin E; Vitamin C in creases iron absorption
Isoniazid	Vitamin B6
Methotrexate	Folic Acid
Methylbromide as preservative	Pantothenic acid
Mineral oil	Vitamins A, E, and K
Neomycin	Vitamin B12
Penicillamine	Vitamin B6
Rancid fats and oils	Vitamin E
Steroids	Vitamin C
Thyroid hormone	Vitamin E

If you have continuing nausea, even when you eat before taking vitamins and nutrients, we advise omitting the zinc. If the nausea goes away after discontinuing the zinc, the dosage of zinc should be halved. Is the small amount tolerable? We advise our patients to cut their dosage of zinc in half, and in half again until they find the dosage they can tolerate. They also divide their dosages between morning and night. If they cannot tolerate zinc at all, they discontinue it. It must be said, though, that we have never had anyone who could not tolerate zinc in minute quantities.

Sometimes, women who have never had menstrual cramps before find that they develop cramps during their periods after they have begun the nutrient program, even if they are having some success with their premenstrual problems. For these women we recommend half an aspirin every day for the three weeks prior to menstruation. Or, we recommend a prostaglandin inhibitor such as ibuprofen, which is very effective for menstrual cramps (sold over-the-counter under the brand names Advil or Nuperin). These prostaglandin inhibitors need only be taken for a day or two while the cramps are present, they can then be discontinued. They have few side effects when taken for such a short period.

Another phenomenon that occurs infrequently after beginning the nutrient program is that the menstrual cycle lengthens. A 28-day cycle, for example, will stretch into a 30- or 31-day cycle. A woman who has had short 20- to 22-day cycles may develop a "normal" 28-day one. Most women consider this a "bonus" of the treatment.

There are few people who cannot tolerate the B vitamins, but every now and then we do come across one. If you decide to take B vitamins but have problems with nausea, lethargy or headache, then decrease your dosage of the vitamin B-complex. See how well your system tolerates the lower dosage (over a period of one to three months), while continuing to take an additional 50 mg of B6 separately.

If you still have difficulty tolerating the B vitamins, check the label on the bottle. What base has been used? Many of the B vitamin pills are yeast-based, but some of the people taking them are intolerant of yeast and yeast products. You may be one of those people. Intolerance to a B vitamin that is yeast-based may indicate a yeast overgrowth problem.

Similarly, a vitamin that is corn-based, which is very common, often causes problems because of unknown allergies to corn. Sensitivity to such a vitamin may indicate an allergy, even if you don't think you have one. People often have allergies to the very foods they think they enjoy the most. Try a B-complex that uses a different base. If you tolerate it well, but did not tolerate the corn-based vitamin, you probably have an allergy to corn. This happens so frequently that we now check the vitamin base whenever a patient comes in with a problem tolerating the B-complexes.

Phony Nutrients

Buying nutrients is a trek into the jungle, where the determined seeker is confronted by an overgrowth of vitamins of varying kinds, brands, dosages, bases, combined ingredients and additives. There are sales, and there are substantial price differences from one brand to another, and from one store to another. Some vitamins are sold only at health food stores, others only at drug stores, still others at grocery stores or specialty stores or through a physician only. Certain vitamins are needlessly expensive, others cost more because they are expensive to produce.

In addition, vitamins contain numerous ingredients that may (or may not) find their way onto the labels. Vitamin manufacturers often list only the active ingredients in their formulations, although the tablets may contain numerous other ingredients like cottonseed oil, sugar, gelatin, food starch, or preservatives such as BHT and BHA. There are fillers and binders, coloring and flavorings. Vitamin C is often passed through corn starch during its processing. Polyvinylpropylone povidone (PVP) is a filler sometimes used to coat the nutrients—but it coats them so well that they pass straight through the body without benefit of first being absorbed. Sugars are added to chewable vitamins to make them palatable (and possibly a source of cavities). Shellacs, waxes, dyes, salt and wheat are also commonplace in our vitamins.

Our general advice about buying vitamins is to check the labels for all ingredients, including the excipient (filler). In addition, check out each brand, each company, as well as you can. The manufacturer's name and where its offices are located are required on vitamin labels. Call the manufacturer directly if you have a question about the ingredients. Ask your doctor or pharmacist to help you with the information. In addition, the Linus Pauling Institute has begun extensive testing of vitamins and nutrients, and will be awarding its own "Seal of Approval" to vitamins after testing. At present there are no federal standards for these supplements.

Vitamin C

The cheapest vitamin C tablet you can buy is probably as good as the most expensive one, so buy the cheap ones. The crystals of vitamin C are often the least expensive form and can be added to orange juice or some other drink.

Vitamin B-Complex

The B-complexes are, however, another story. A low-cost vitamin B-complex may be a low-quality one. This is partially because the B vitamins must be present in a particular ratio to be of optimal use (see page 99). Some of the B vitamins cost much more than others, and often a manufacturer will include great quantities of the less expensive Bs.

How can you tell whether or not they are present in the correct proportions? First of all, look at the list of ingredients and their quantities. Then look into the reputation of the manufacturer. Check with your local pharmacist, doctor, or health food store.

Another important thing to look for is what the vitamin B is made from. What base has been used? Most B vitamins are based on yeast, a very cheap, very good source. But yeast is often the cause of a host of other problems, mostly stemming from an intestinal yeast overgrowth, but also due to allergic reactions. Also, yeast can exacerbate all of the problems of premenstrual syndrome, as we explain later on. The problem of intestinal yeast overgrowth is beginning to get widespread attention, and some doctors are now advising their patients to stop taking vitamins that have a yeast base—most often found in B vitamin pills. In addition, people who have allergies to rice, corn or wheat should be sure to check the label to see whether the vitamins are based on any of these substances.

Instead of taking vitamins that are yeast- or rice-based (the two most common bases), we recommend hypoallergenic B complexes. These tend to cost more, but we feel they are worth it because you can be sure of what you are getting—and you can be fairly sure you are not going to be getting more problems than you are solving.

OTHER NUTRIENTS

Zinc is inexpensive and readily available. A calcium-magnesium supplement is also standard.

Vitamins will generally keep, so it is possible to buy them in large quantities. However, when you are in the initial phase of experimenting with dosages, we recommend purchasing the vitamins and nutrients in small quantities. Should there be problems with a particular nutrient, or a particular brand or dosage, the program can easily be altered.

Evening Primrose Oil

Evening primrose oil has a very distinct odor and taste. Some people find it pleasant, others do not. It does not have a "rosy" taste or smell. Much of the "primrose oil" on the market today, especially those brands with a pronounced rosy aroma or taste, are not evening primrose oil and do not contain gammalinolenic acid, the active ingredient of evening primrose oil. Without the gammalinolenic acid, you might as well be taking a placebo. An "evening primrose oil" without this active incredient is not able to enhance the formation of prostaglandin E-1. These kinds of primrose oil are either the result of a mistake in the manufacturing process, or they are an outright phony product.

We have been surprised by a number of women who, after having immediate success on the nutrient program, found that their old symptoms returned. "I'm doing everything just the same . . . it simply isn't working anymore," they would tell us. At first we were terriby concerned and confused. Why weren't they better? What had happened? What had changed? We quizzed them on everything—their diet, their nutrient dosages, their diary-keeping—only to find that the brand of primrose oil they were using was of dubious quality. Usually, they had switched to a capsule that was being offered at a low price from a discount service. Sometimes they had switched simply because a certain brand was sold at a convenient pharmacy or health food store. In every case, when they substituted a tested brand for whatever they had been taking, their symptoms disappeared immediately and they returned to good health. The effective ingredient, gammalinolenic acid, must be present in sufficient quantities to be effective. Otherwise, it is a waste of money.

EXERCISE   Consistent exercise, always an important aspect of general health, is especially necessary for women trying to rid themselves of PMS. Exercise improves cardio-vascular status and significantly reduces the amount of stress on the system. It assists the body's metabolic processes, allowing it to better use nutritional supplements, medication and foods. Dosages of supplements and medicines can be reduced for people who exercise regularly.

Before you start an exercise program get a medical evaluation and physical examination—particularly if you have any doubts about your general health.

We suggest a slow start with a steady build-up. If you are too tired to exercise, start with just a few minutes per day. If you think you don't have enough time to exercise, then you probably really need to. If you've ever stuck to an exercise routine, you already know that it will give you extra energy and, consequently, extra time. People who have trouble mustering the energy to exercise are usually nutritionally deficient and their bodies are working under a handicap. As you handle your nutritional problems, it may become easier to put the time aside for an exercise program.

Develop a long-term program that includes aerobic exercise as well as stretching and muscle-building exercises. Choose exercises that you can do regularly, whether at home or away. Plan for exercise all year long, in spite of changing weather conditions.

Try to exercise in the morning, as this will give you added lift and help in waking up. Have your exercise area ready, or easy to clear out every day. Minimize the hurdles that lie in the way of regular exercise by setting up an area with enough room to exercise. Equip yourself with a cassette tape player if you want to exercise to music. In fact, a tape with directions and music can shape your exercise time into a pleasant ritual that you never skimp on.

Basic Exercise Program

On the first day of your exercise program do no more than 10 to 15 seconds of calisthenic exercises (such as jumping jacks), and no more than one minute of gentle running, bicycling or swimming. On the following two or three days, repeat Day 1. On Day 4, increase each section gradually by adding 10 seconds to each calisthenic exercise and doing aerobics for up to 2 minutes. On Days 5 and 6, repeat Day 4. On Day 7 and after, add a little extra time to each exercise. Move up gradually to 5 minutes a day of calisthenics and 10 minutes of aerobics. Resist the impulse to overdo it, and resist the impulse to skip the whole thing.

Can you take your pulse? With the third and fourth fingers of one hand, find the pulse in your opposite wrist. Count the number of pulse beats during a 60-second interval. If you count more than 120 or 130 after exercising, you may be working your body too strenuously and may even be doing yourself harm. Under 100 or 110 means that you are not exerting yourself enough. After two months of exercise, bring your rate higher, to 140 or 150 after five minutes of exercise. Keep it there for about ten minutes, then gradually wind down. Take several minutes for winding down. Never exceed 160 beats per minute unless you consult a physician.

CALIS-THENICS

Begin slowly, doing each excercise once. Increase each movement series every day until you reach a five-minute total. Design your own program, leaving out or changing any exercises that aren't suited to your physical condition or that are painful. Experiment with these exercises as energy boosters for those odd times of the day when you need a lift.

Sit Ups

Use either the knees-up or the legs-flat-on-the-floor method. Try holding your head a few inches off the ground for several seconds at a time.

Knee Bends

Keep your shoulders back, your hands on your hips, and your back straight.

Head Rolls   In a standing position, allow your head to drop forward, then roll it smoothly to the left, the back, the right, returning to the front in a circle. Then reverse directions.

Arm Circles   Extend your arms sideways, while you are standing. Keeping your arms straight, move your arms in a circular motion, making five small circles, then five large circles. Reverse directions.

Toe-Touching   From a sitting position, with your legs stretched out in front, bend your trunk and reach for your toes. Reach as far as you can without straining. If you can't touch your toes now, you'll be able to do so in a week, or in a month, or a few months.

Side Bends   From a standing position, bend sideways to the right as far as you can without straining. Hold this position for a count of five. Return to an upright position and repeat to the left side.

Arm Twists   In a standing position, extend your arms sideways. Without moving your feet, twist your body to the left as far as you can without straining. Repeat in the opposite direction.

Reach-Out   From a standing position, bend at the waist with your back straight. Bend at the waist and reach forward with your arms, always keeping your back straight. You should look like an L on its side. Let your arms drop, and repeat.

Knee Ups	In a standing position, bring your left knee up to your chest. Help it up with your hands. Return it to the ground, and repeat the motion with your right knee.
Leg Lifts	Lie on your side using one hand to support your head and the other to balance yourself on the floor. Lift one leg as far towards the ceiling as you can without straining. Repeat three times, then change sides.
AEROBICS	Aerobic exercise basically involves increasing your heart rate by running, hopping, jumping, dancing, kicking, swimming, biking, etc. The idea is to raise your body's metabolism to a higher-than-usual level and to maintain that level for an extended period.
	Set an ultimate goal of getting your pulse rate up to 140 beats per minute for 20 to 30 minutes, but start at no more than 3 or 4 minutes. Take at least 10 weeks to reach this goal; it may take as many as 20 weeks or more. When you have reached your goal, do aerobic exercising for half an hour, three to six times a week.
Jogging	Start slowly by simply walking. Then try a combination of walking and jogging, mostly walking. Build this up over time, increasing the amount of jogging to the full 30-minute duration. First, walk a quarter of a mile. Then try half a mile, three-quarters of a mile, then a mile. Try walking for three-quarters of a mile and jogging for the last quarter. Then add 30 seconds or less per day of actual running time until you are running for 30 minutes without straining or gasping for air.
	If you experience any physical problems while following this plan, stop until you have recovered. Wait five days and then begin again, going half as fast as you did before. If the problem recurs, see your physician

for a re-evaluation. If you experience upper chest or left arm pain, severe dizziness or fainting feelings while exercising, see your doctor before continuing.

Cycling

Begin with 30 seconds on the exercycle or the equivalent on the bicycle, depending on the terrain. Take your pulse and record it. Increase your time by 30 seconds each day for 10 days, or the equivalent. Increase your time until you can do 30 minutes, three to six times per week, with a pulse rate of 120 to 140.

Swimming

Find a place where you can swim laps. Start with one lap, then gradually increase the number of laps, going at increments of 30 seconds or less per day, until you are swimming for at least 5 minutes. Check your pulse. Increase your time gradually, by 30 seconds or less each day, until you reach 30 minutes. Then, work at getting your pulse in the 120 to 140 range, and keeping it there while you swim. Swim for half an hour three times a week.

6

WHAT TO EXPECT

After someone with PMS has been taking the nutrients for about six months, they often find that they can—and should—decrease their dosage. They have been providing their system with things that were previously deficient, but now their bodies are back to running efficiently. As the body runs more and more efficiently, it needs less replenishment, partially because it is not as susceptible to biochemical stress as before, not as needy in general. In addition, the body begins to absorb the nutrients more efficiently. With respect to the nutrients that can be stored in the body, higher doses are often needed at first. As the empty body reservoirs are filled up, much lower regular doses are required to keep the reservoirs topped up.

Sometimes, after five to seven months of doing very well on a particular dosage of nutrients, minor problems might occur. Our suggestion if this happens is usually to first reduce the dosage. Start by cutting it in half, or stretching it out over a longer period of time. Thus, instead of increasing the dosage after one week, increase it after ten days so that there is less of a build-up in the system.

In short, the process depends on the individual. A person with PMS should experience some relief within the first two months of starting the nutrient program. Usually, the symptoms of PMS are brought well under control within six months and the dosages of optimal efficiency have been found. After that, a woman might stay on a particular dosage and program for three to nine months, and may subsequently find that she wants to cut back somewhat on the nutrient supplement dosages. Others may decide to remain with exactly the same program.

The typical patient comes to us saying, "I can't stand the way I am. I just can't go on this way. If I just didn't feel *quite* so awful part of every month."

We admit that the first month may not bring any great changes—no miracles, no fabulous cures. What we are looking for, we remind them, is a percentage of change. We look for a significant percentage of improvement in the first month. For instance, headaches for only two days instead of four, or bloating four pounds instead of six. Other typical first-month responses are mood swings that are not quite as pronounced as before, or hostility that lasts only three days instead of five.

Each time we point out these facts, there is a great sigh of relief and the patient says that it sounds terrific. We develop a nutrient program for her to begin right away. Several weeks later, after her next premenstrual time, we ask how it went.

"Not very well," she says. "I still had some symptoms. I bloated up a pound and I yelled at my children several times. I got ticked off at some small, unimportant things."

We'll sometimes find there may even be a 50 or 60 percent improvement. The fact is, *the symptoms of PMS do not disappear in the first month for 95 percent of afflicted women.* There is usually some improvement, but it is not as noticeable as it will be later.

Some improvement in the first month is encouraging and indicates that the problem can be dealt with successfully on a nutritional basis; complete success is rarely instantaneous. Primrose oil and vitamin therapy is not always dramatic; it pains us to see a woman getting upset and discouraged because she is not instantly cured. We now emphasize to our patients that the changes they undergo may be gradual.

THE TIMETABLE

The First Month

Seventy percent of women with PMS show an improvement of between 20 and 80 percent during the first month of primrose oil and nutrient supplementation. If there is no improvement, or very minimal improvement during the first month, we consider other approaches. Most commonly we look at vitamin malabsorption, a deficiency of vitamin B_{12}, yeast overgrowth, and allergies. (We will explain each of these and what to do about them in the next chapter.)

The Second Month

Month 2 generally brings a greater improvement— about 40 to 50 percent for most women.

The Third Month

Month 3 often brings a contradictory phenomenon, with the body either stabilizing or experiencing a setback. Setbacks are surprising and distressing for most women, especially for those to whom the second month brought significant relief. If this relapse is a significant one, we alter the primrose oil dosage as follows.

If a PMS problem of lethargy or headache resurfaces during Month 3, when a low dosage of primrose oil is being taken, then we increase the dosage to about 4 or 5 capsules a day.

If a person finds herself lethargic and/or headachy, and if she is already on a high dosage of primrose oil, then we decrease the dosage slightly.

The Fourth Month

Month 4 is usually relatively good. The body is getting used to the new balance of essential fatty acids and prostaglandins. Beyond the fourth month, things should continue to improve steadily.

At any time, however, it is possible that fewer nutrients will be sufficient. Our patients often decrease the dosage a little bit every day after about six months of stabilization. We prefer this to skipping dosages, but we believe that every individual should experiment to find how she can best meet her own needs. Alternatively, the program can be stopped altogether, to be resumed if the symptoms of PMS return.

FINE TUNING

It is advisable to try different amounts of the nutrients, experimenting with optimal dosages of each nutrient and what each nutrient does. For instance, a woman who has acne that does not improve by the second month may find that increasing her dosage of zinc up to 30 mg per day is helpful.

Only one nutrient should ever be changed at a time, so that all changes can be readily observed. Any woman who decides to develop her own nutrient program will have to become her own detective. Her most helpful tool will be the diary.

The success rate for nutrients plus primrose oil as we've outlined it has been about 70 percent. With the addition of treatment for allergies and *Candida albicans* overgrowth, the success rate has been about 85 percent overall. We have also used tiny amounts of extract of progesterone to stimulate the hormonal system of some patients, and this additional technique has brought the success rate up still further.

In a British study, Michael Brush, M.D., gave primrose oil to 70 women who had not responded to other PMS treatment. Sixty percent of these problem patients derived "major relief" from primrose oil, 20 percent had "moderate relief," and 20 percent reported "no change." Theoretically, if the group had been an average mix of premenstrual sufferers, the positive results would have been even higher. Most of the trials used a standard dosage of six to eight capsules of primrose oil per day, with no additional nutrients. We feel that an individually tailored dosage of evening primrose oil plus additional nutrients will give optimal results. One tablespoon per day of uncooked, unprocessed, pressed safflower oil has a 20 percent success rate.

The biggest problem is discouragement. Women often get discouraged if they take vitamins and nutrients for a few weeks only to find, when their pre-time comes, that they are still plagued with symptoms of PMS. PMS is not going to go away in the first month. That's all there is to it. You have to be aware—constantly—that PMS involves a process that is ongoing all month long, and it takes time to regulate it. Although we may be acutely aware of a prostaglandin imbalance for only a few days out of the month, it is a month-long process that builds up.

It is their commitment to handling their PMS that carries people through treatment. You can't try a nutrient program on for size, you can't check it out for a few days and then drop it. You can't dabble with it for a week to "see what happens." Even if it doesn't solve your problems in the first month, you have not fully tried it unless you keep going, and keep watching how your body is working. You should see some relief the first month, but it may not be enough to keep disappointment away.

7

PATIENTS
WITH PROBLEMS

What do we do when a clear-cut case of PMS does not respond to the nutrient program or when the response is inadequate? What are the most common underlying reasons?

VITAMIN MAL-ABSORPTION

One possible problem is a vitamin B_{12} deficiency. When vitamin B_{12} was first discovered, it was hailed as a cure-all and used to treat nearly every symptom in the medical books. If someone had a headache, they were given a shot of vitamin B_{12}. If it was a cold, a vitamin B_{12} shot would turn it around. If it was the flu, B_{12} was prescribed. It was the most over-used vitamin in the world. Then the medical community went to the opposite extreme and stopped using vitamin B_{12} injections entirely. Now it is used infrequently, for specific B_{12} deficiencies.

We feel there is a middle ground and that extra vitamin B_{12} is needed by many of the women who suffer from premenstrual syndrome. As mentioned earlier, the B vitamins, sometimes referred to as the "energy vitamins," are necessary for metabolism as a whole to function properly. In addition, the B vitamins must be present in certain proportions. If B_{12} is not present, or is not being absorbed properly, the system falls into an imbalance that, in itself, can lead to physical and/or psychological problems. In addition, we have found that there is no "normal" level of B_{12} that is right for everyone.

When someone with PMS does not respond to the nutrients, we sometimes try to remedy the situation with additional vitamin B_{12}, even if blood tests show a "normal" B_{12} level. The way we see it, the normal range for B_{12} is actually a very wide one that encompasses many different levels. Although you may have a B_{12} level of 450 or 500, which is considered normal, you may need a 900 level to function at your best. We assume that everyone has different needs, and that even if they have a "normal" level of B_{12}, there is a possibility that they may need supplementation.

Vitamin B_{12} is available in the diet only through meat, which makes supplementation particularly important for vegetarians. (It raises the question, however, of whether vegetarians are willing to use vitamins derived from animals.) In addition, vitamin B_{12} cannot be metabolized without a substance called the *intrinsic factor* (a substance in the lining of the stomach). Some people are born without this intrinsic factor, and have difficulty metabolizing vitamin B_{12} properly; they usually need regular supplementation.

CASE HISTORY: Sarah S.

Sarah S. had a huge problem with low energy, especially during her pre-time. She was also depressed and found that, premenstrually, she suffered from a loss of motivation. Sarah taught at an elementary school and was disturbed when she did not have her usual tolerance for and patience with the children. She began the nutrient program, but did not respond well. Her depression was only slightly better, but her energy level remained low. She was very discouraged. Discussing her history in a little more detail with her, we discovered that her mother had had a problem with anemia and had taken B12 injections for years. As soon as we tried B12 with Sarah, she felt much better.

The B12 injection did not clear up the premenstrual syndrome problems, but it helped Sarah's energy level and general feeling of health. She could feel the difference, and she could tell whenever the B12 wore off. When she resumed taking nutrients—along with regular B12 injections—Sarah's pre-period problems virtually disappeared. The B12 metabolism process had been interfering with her ability to use the other nutrients, and once the B12 deficiency was taken care of, Sarah was able to absorb the other nutrients efficiently.

MENSTRUAL CRAMPS

Sometimes, menstrual cramps can cause discomfort for the first, second, or third day of menses. Aspirin or a prostaglandin inhibitor, ibuprofen (trade names are Advil, Nuprin, Anaprox, and Motrin) can often alleviate much of the cramping and discomfort.

Aspirin is best taken as half a tablet daily for the three weeks prior to menstruation. Ibuprofen should be taken every four to six hours—one or two tablets at a time—to 1200 mg in a twenty-four hour period. Advil and Nuprin (over-the-counter, non-prescription medication) both contain 200 mg of ibuprofen per tablet, while Motrin (by prescription) has two sizes, 300 mg (white) or 400 mg (orange).

CASE HISTORY: Rose M.

Rose M. came to us with severe PMS problems, which she had had ever since she first got her period at age 12. They were bad enough, she told us, to have hindered her noticeably in school because she was unable to concentrate. Rose was 25 years old, recently married, and working as a salesperson when we first met her. She had terrible headaches, low energy, depression, irritability, and she fought incessantly with her husband during her premenstrual time. Finally, she suffered from severe menstrual cramps.

Rose's mother heard about us through a friend and made an appointment for her daughter, who was reluctant to come in. We started her slowly on a regimen of primrose oil and co-factor vitamins geared to her symptoms. It took several months, but we figured out a program that handled her pre-time quite well. She had more energy, was less irritable, fought less with her husband and co-workers, and generally felt better.

"I used to feel like I was a split personality, but now I'm just one person," she was fond of saying. Her menstrual cramps, however, persisted. (Cramps of this magnitude are called dysmenorrhea.) They could be devastating, and frequently made it impossible for her to go to work. We put her on 300 mg of prostaglandin inhibitor Motrin at the onset of cramping, and three more capsules at two-hour intervals. Within twenty minutes of taking the first anti-prostaglandin, the cramps were gone. Her pre-period and menstrual problems are no longer an issue in her life. Rose continues to take the nutrients, at a lower dosage than before, and she takes Motrin whenever she is troubled by menstrual cramps.

PROLONGED MENSTRUAL CYCLE

A rather unusual problem is prolonged cycle, where the menstrual cycle sometimes drags on for as many as fifty or sixty days. Premenstrual signs may begin on Day 21, for instance, but drag on until Day 42. The cycle can be brought back to normal by discontinuing the primrose oil two days before the period would normally be expectd to begin. Then, the primrose oil is resumed after the menstrual flow stops. This action of primrose oil is effective only when the periods are extremely lengthy. Normal cycles are not affected, and discontinuing primrose oil will not bring on the menstrual flow in women with normal cycles. The primrose oil seems to have a normalizing effect on cycle length, bringing both shorter cycles of 20–22 days and longer cycles of 40–60 days back into the normal range of 28–30 days.

CASE HISTORY: Rachel M.

Rachel M. had quite a few problems associated with her period, including an extended cycle. She was extremely irregular; sometimes her cycle was forty days, sometimes fifty. She would get premenstrual on Day 27 or so, and her pre-time would stretch out miserably. She had emotional outbursts as well as bloating problems. We put her on the nutrient program and added diuretics because her bloating was extreme and debilitating. The bloating was brought under control and the emotional components improved, but the periods were still extended and irregular. So Rachel stopped taking the primrose oil on Day 28, two days before she thought she should be getting her period. (She felt that her normal cycle was 30 days.) To her delight, her cycle stablilized after a few months at around a 30-day cycle.

Rachel is doing well now, and has made several major changes in her life "because I'm feeling so much better . . . I have the energy now to change things, to say 'No, I want my life to be different.' " She is a more lively, vibrant, and happy person now that menstruation is no longer a factor in her personality.

BLOATING

Diuretics used to be the automatic prescription for bloating associated with premenstrual syndrome. It was even thought that if bloating was brought under control, all other manifestations of PMS would miraculously disappear. Why? It was thought that if bloating could be controlled, then the patient would feel more attractive, and therefore less depressed, irritable, and hostile—nor would she get acne. Women who had premenstrual bloating problems were routinely given diuretics.

Of course, that was erroneous thinking. Often, while diuretics reduced bloating, they made psychological symptoms worse. Furthermore, to control bloating, lifestyle and nutritional approaches are usually sufficient. We use diuretics only if all else fails.

The first step we take is to restrict salt in the diet. North Americans eat an average of 15 pounds (6.75 kg) of salt a year, which breaks down to about 3 teaspoons (15 mL) a day; we require only about one-tenth of a teaspoon of salt a day. Many women find they crave salt during the premenstrual time, which increases the swelling of tissues and bloating problems. Although it is difficult to completely avoid sodium, as it is present in almost all processed foods, baked goods, dairy products, canned foods, drugs, and even frozen vegetables, all efforts should be made to restrict it for ten days prior to menstruation if bloating is a problem. (See the chart on the next page for the sodium content of common foods.)

Read the label on all processed foods and eliminate those with high salt content, such as packaged cold cereals, canned soups, canned vegetables, butter and margarine, salad dressings, and cookies and desserts.

Call your local water district to find out the sodium content of your water, which is often very high. Some water filters can remove sodium when placed on your faucet. An ion-exchanger will also remove sodium.

Avoid antacids, laxatives and cough preparations that contain salt. Eat fresh foods, cooked from scratch without added salt. Use herbs and spices that do not contain salt. Throw away your table salt shaker. By eliminating or restricting your salt intake, as well as minimizing premenstrual bloating, you will also be

SODIUM CONTENT OF SELECTED FOODS[8]

Food	Mg Sodium Content
chicken, 2 pieces, roasted	57
Pepperidge Farm white bread, slice	117
milk, 8 oz.	130
Planter's Cocktail Peanuts, 1 oz.	132
Heinz Tomato Catsup, 1 tbsp.	154
Skippy Creamy Peanut Butter, 2 tbsp.	167
Lay's Potato Chips, 14 chips	191
Kraft American Singles Cheese Food, 1 slice	238
Kellogg's Corn Flakes, 1 oz.	260
Campbell's Tomato Juice, 6 oz.	292
Oscar Mayer Bacon, 3 slices	302
Wishbone Italian Dressing	315
Del Monte Sweet Peas, drained, 5 ¼ oz.	349
flounder, broiled filets, 2 oz.	355
chuck steak,cooked, lean, 8.4 oz.	381
Jell-O Chocolate Flavor Instant Pudding and Pie Filling, .5 cup	404
Breakstone's Lowfat Cottage Cheese, 4 oz.	435
Bumble Bee Brand Albacore Chunk White Tuna, drained, 3 ¼ oz.	628
Oscar Mayer Bologna, 3 slices	672
Herb-Ox Instant Broth and Seasoning Beef Flavored, 1 packet	818
Campbell's Beans & Franks, 8 oz.	958
Heinz Dill Pickles, 1 large	1137
Swanson Fried Chicken Dinner, 1 dinner	1152
Chef Boyardee Beefaroni, 7.5 oz.	1186
Big Mac, 1	1510

lowering your risk of high blood pressure and hypertension, a major cause of death in North America today.

In addition to restricted salt, we increase vitamin B6 (pyridoxine) to about 200 mg a day to treat bloating problems. Pyridoxine is known as a natural diuretic. It helps maintain chemical balances in the tissues and helps to regulate the excretion of water. Pyridoxine is found naturally in fish (herring, salmon, mackerel, and tuna), meats (especially liver), peanuts, molasses, spinach, soybeans, legumes, bananas, whole grains, yams, and walnuts. We do not recommend that people take large dosages of pyridoxine for more than several days in a row, as it may, paradoxically, increase the body's needs for the vitamin. We also encourage eating fresh grapefruit, which acts as a natural diuretic.

If bloating continues to be a problem, then we will use a diuretic for a two- to three-day period (or less). We prescribe a low dosage, taken in the morning and used in conjunction with the nutrients. Generally, we favor Hydrodiuril or Aldactone. However, Hydrodiuril depletes potassium, and anyone taking it must eat plenty of potassium. Good sources of potassium are tomato juice, bananas, citrus juices, wheat germ, beans, lentils, nuts, dates, prunes, and green, leafy vegetables. Aldactone is potassium-sparing; women using it need not increase their potassium intake.

CANDIDA ALBICANS

A large number of women who have premenstrual syndrome also have allergies and/or an overgrowth of *Candida albicans* yeast in the intestine. Both of these underlying conditions can exaggerate the symptoms of premenstrual syndrome and can cause them to last throughout the month, though they will be more intense during the pre-time.

Candida albicans is normally present in small quantities in our intestines, but under certain circumstances, a situation can occur in which there is an overgrowth. "If we were to try in one simple sentence to describe the clinical picture most suggestive of this condition," writes Dr. C. Orion Truss, who is largely responsible for the increasing public awareness of this condition through his book, *The Missing Diagnosis*, "it would be that of a woman between puberty and menopause who has begun having vaginal symptoms (discharge, itching, or both) and/or bowel symptoms (constipation or diarrhea, excess gas, abdominal distention and discomfort), abnormalities of the menstrual cycle and flow, absent or diminished libido, and a personality change characterized by abnormal emotions (depression, extreme irritability, anxiety, crying), deterioration in intellectual function (concentration, memory, reasoning), and a destructive loss of self-confidence so severe that it may result in her inability to cope with even the simplest problem." It should be noted that men and children can be similarly affected by yeast overgrowth, although it is more commonly present in women.

There are several problems inherent in trying to make a diagnosis of *Candida*. One of them is the ubiquitous presence of the yeast bacteria under normal circumstances, combined with the fact that our lab tests do not measure the quantitative presence of yeast adequately. While most mainstream physicians do recognize intestinal yeast as a medical problem, they tend to bypass its presence unless it is at its most severe, debilitating form—an extreme that most people never reach. Thus, most doctors see *Candida* overgrowth as an extremely rare disease, although we believe that it is frequently at the crux of their patients' problems.

In fact, intestinal yeast is not rare at all. We see a tremendous amount of it, as do our colleagues all over the country. The markers for intestinal yeast problems are:

- history of thrush as an infant
- a history of the adult equivalent of thrush, a yeast infection in the mouth
- a history of vaginal infections and cystitis
- regular, frequent or extensive use of antibiotics at any time during the patient's past
- use of birth control pills at any time during the patient's past
- bowel problems, including alternating constipation and diarrhea, bloating or distention (not limited to, but including premenstrually)
- difficulty getting pregnant
- problems with post-partum depression, especially when it lingers on

In addition, pregnancy itself can encourage an overgrowth of yeast organisms. Like birth control pills, pregnancy alters the acid balance of the vaginal tract and creates an environment that is hospitable to yeast overgrowth. (It seems that the yeast creates more acidity in the vaginal tract, which may explain why women with yeast overgrowth problems so often have trouble getting pregnant. The sperm may not be able to survive the acidity created by the yeast. This difficulty usually disappears when the *Candida* infection is taken care of.)

If a woman has had this sort of history and has experienced emotional problems—mood swings, fatigue and loss of motivation, or diminished sex drive—for a long period of time, we immediately suspect intestinal yeast. Birth control pills and antibiotics in the history are particularly important, as both destroy the natural flora of the intestines and create a climate that is conducive to the growth and multiplication of yeast cells. Yeast overgrowth often follows antibiotic use, and anyone taking antibiotics should also eat acidophillus yogurt (yogurt with an active culture) to help maintain the balance of intestinal bacteria.

As yeast overgrowth intensifies, the yeast organisms and their by-products begin to interfere with various systems of the body. One of the first areas to be affected is the gastrointestinal tract and bowels. This causes the constipation and bloating that so commonly plague women. Vaginal infections are also extremely common. The yeast also reaches various systems of the body, and yeast overgrowth can also effect the reproductive system itself, contributing to, or even causing premenstrual syndrome.

When we suspect a *Candida* problem, we put the patient on the nutrient program as usual, but we also immediately start her on Nystatin, a medication that kills yeast, or a new, non-medication formula called Capristatin (an essential fatty acid-based substance).

Nystatin works only on yeast cells; it does not dissolve in water. Even when large amounts of Nyastatin are swallowed, very little of it gets into the blood stream. Thus it is quite different from most medications, some of which act by moving through the blood stream. It has almost no toxicity and, says the *Physician's Desk Reference (PDR)*, "Nystatin is virtually nontoxic and nonsensitizing and is well tolerated by all age groups, even on prolonged administration." Nystatin is available by prescription only.

If a person does not have a yeast problem and takes Nystatin, there is no noticeable effect. We know there is a yeast problem when the Nystatin attacks yeast cells and toxins are released in the process. The toxins often cause a temporary return of symptoms, called the Herxheimer Reaction, and this phenomenon lasts from an hour to several days or even longer. Because it can be quite severe, with discomfort from aching, bloating, headache stuffiness or worsening of whatever problems the patient originally sought help for, we generally start of with a very low dosage, a toothpick "dot" of the powder. (One-eighth of a teaspoon is equal to 500,000 units.) After we see how well the patient tolerates such a low dosage, we work up to a higher one. Generally, using Nystatin along with the nutrient program, avoidance of yeast foods, and maintaining only a low level of carbohydrates in the diet, provide significant relief from premenstrual syndrome.

We have recently begun to use a nutrient preparation, Capristatin, in the treatment of intestinal yeast problems. Capristatin can be as effective as Nystatin, and may have certain advantages. Capristatin is a nutrient (a saturated fatty acid), not a medication. It is also a broad-spectrum fungicide that destroys the *Candida* strain throughout the body. Capristatin seems to have fewer side effects associated with it, although any antifungal preparation can produce yeast die-off symptoms. Capristatin should only be used as part of an antifungal program and should be administered under the supervision of a physician.

To avoid yeast in the diet, use a low-mold, low-carbohydrate diet. Molds are closely related to *Candida*, and carbohydrates provide a ready medium for yeast growth. People who suspect that they have a *Candida* problem should go on a low-mold, low-carbohydrate diet for one week and observe whether or not they feel better. Foods to be avoided include sugary foods of all kinds, such as candies, cakes, ice cream, soft drinks, honey, maple syrup, corn syrup, and carob; yeast-containing foods, such as mushrooms, bakery products made with yeast, wines, beer and other fermented beverages, cheese, vinegars; dried fruits, melons, juices; and vitamin supplements that are yeast-based. Emphasized are low carbohydrate vegetables such as lettuce, spinach, broccoli, squash, cauliflower, cucumbers and asparagus, and high-protein foods such as fish, lean meats, nuts and eggs.

In addition, moldy places such as damp basements should be avoided.

A way to think of the *Candida* problem is that it ofen results from taking antibiotics. Antibiotics disrupt the normal flora in the large intestine because they kill the bacteria ordinarily present. When antibiotics first came into use, the medical profession's approach was that if they helped people fight off a disease, then killing bacteria in the intestinal tract was fine. But it is now known that for the absorption of many of the B vitamins, and probably many other substances, those intestinal bacteria are necessary. Some vitamins are actually made in the intestinal bacteria. Certain vitamins are not absorbed earlier in the digestive process; they must be broken down by the normal intestinal bacteria. But when antibiotics destroy these particular bacteria, the *Candida* thrive in their stead.

Once the *Candida* yeast has established itself, the bacteria do not seem to be able to make a comeback and repopulate to their normal levels. Eventually, this affects the hormone regulation system and contributes to premenstrual discomfort. Finally, it is important to note that there seems to be a direct connection between the yeast and the immune response system, including allergies, and when we treat someone for a yeast infection, we very often find that their allergies clear up.

CASE HISTORY: Silvia R.

Sylvia R. came to us because of severe PMS problems. She experienced mood changes, irritability, crying, and repeated episodes of "flying off the handle." Furthermore, she had cramping, some bloating, and breast tenderness for about ten days before her period. During the premenstrual time, she told us, she was completely unpredictable.

"I have no idea how I'll react to something," she complained. "Someone can say something to me and I'll get completely hysterical. I cry, I carry on, I get furious." Innocent remarks like "That's a nice blouse, Sylvia. I've always liked it on you," would trigger a violent reaction and feelings of "devastation." " 'I'm wearing the same old rag again,' I would think, 'and people recognize it. They see it all the time, they're tired of seeing it.' "

Sylvia adapted well to the nutrient program, deriving about 50 to 60 percent relief. However, the crying spells and cravings for heavy breads and cheeses persisted. After about three and a half months, she felt she was not going to get further relief from the nutrient program.

Knowing that Sylvia had a history of antibiotic use as a teenager (to clear up an acne problem), and that she had been on birth control pills for several months during her late teens, we began to suspect a yeast problem. Then she told us that she had had frequent problems with diarrhea in the past, which convinced us to try Nystatin. She also began a low-mold, low-carbohydrate diet.

Within two months, most of her remaining symptoms had cleared up. She stayed on the Nystatin for about six months, and then went off it. Gradually, she began to reintroduce small amounts of carbohydrates into her diet, and found she could handle them well. If she has a return of symptoms, she will go back to the Nystatin and the low-mold, low-carbohydrate diet until she gets relief.

ALLERGIES   Allergies can also have a profound effect on premenstrual syndrome, and, as has become increasingly apparent as we work with allergies, they play an integral role in how we feel physically, intellectually, and emotionally. It seems that people today are becoming allergic or sensitive to the air we breathe and the food we eat, to plastics and perfumes, gas and diesel fumes, to rice and eggs, milk, mold, pollen and dust. It is no longer merely our dogs and cats who bring out allergic reactions; it is the furniture we sit on and the cups we drink from.

People with PMS are also often atopic, that is they come from families whose members are unusually suscepti- ble to allergies, allergic rhinitis, asthma, and eczema.

Theoretically, it may be that our environment is evolv- ing faster than our bodies are able to adapt. We haven't adjusted to the changes in nutrition or to the highly chemicallized environment that we live in. As a result, the immune system—which determines what is accept- able, and what is not—is overloaded with unknown substances. It is proving inadequate to the task of deal- ing with all of these foreign substances.

If we suspect that a person has allergies (because of their clinical history and their responses on the allergy questionnaire), we begin to test for specific allergens. We also begin the nutrient program.

First, we test for the most common chemical sensitiv- ities, such as sensitivity to formaldehyde (present in nearly every man-made product in our homes and cars), molds, and tobacco smoke. We test for wheat, milk, eggs, yeast, peanut butter, corn, chocolate and sugar— the most common food allergies. Then we test for substances that are suspected of being particularly prob- lematic for the individual. We also test for the female hormones—progesterone, estrogen, and lutenizing hormone. Some women have a sensitivity to these hormones, and can get relief by taking hormonal ex- tract injections during the premenstrual time.

If the person tested shows a reaction to any of the above tests—usually a headache, hostility, exhaustion, hives, or a very enlarged wheal where the test was made—we give neutralization protection from the specific substance. Our method of neutralization is related to that of the clinical ecologists, a branch of allergy specialists who use a very diluted extract of the substance injected just under the skin.

Another way to find out whether you have food allergies is called "The Challenge." First, completely remove a possibly suspect food from your diet for five days. For instance, you might remove wheat—and that includes breads, cakes, cookies, gravies that are made from flour, candies, cereals, puddings, etc. It takes about three days for a food to leave your system; in five days, you can be pretty sure that the substance has been eliminated. Observe yourself carefully. Have you experienced any withdrawal symptoms? Do you feel worse? Do you feel better? After five days of abstinence, eat the targeted food. "Challenge" it by eating twice as much as usual. Watch yourself for reactions. Typical reactions are sleepiness, stuffiness, headache, cramps, tingling hands and feet, hostility, and crabbiness. If you have a reaction, then you probably have a hidden allergy.

Finally, it is possible to get a sense of whether you're allergic to something by taking Alka Seltzer Gold (without aspirin) after eating a particular food. Alka Seltzer Gold contains potassium and sodium bicarbonate, and acts as a neutralizer for many food allergies. If you feel better after taking Alka Seltzer Gold, consider the possibility that you are allergic to something you have eaten.

CASE HISTORY: Shelley R.

Premenstrual time for Shelley R. was usually a time of throwing coffee pots and experiencing a general loss of control. At the same time, she would become terribly frustrated at her own behavior—an awareness that made the situation even worse. She knew her reactions were inappropriate, but she couldn't seem to control herself. Shelley never hurt anybody, but she got very depressed. She was also overly conscious of her weight, admittedly on the high side. During her pre-time, however, Shelley would decide that she was as big as a house. Finally, she also suffered from migraine headaches.

It was clear from Shelley's evaluation that PMS was a problem, but that there might also be food and environmental allergies. We found through testing that she was allergic to oats, corn, wheat, milk, chlorine, and alcohol. Neutralizing her to these things caused a dramatic turn-around. She reported that she was finally in control again.

CASE HISTORY: Kim M.

Kim and her husband had read about us in the newspaper and came to our offices because Kim had problems that seemed to be premenstrually related. Hallucinations and severe anxiety had grown to the point where they interfered grotesquely with her life.

We tried everything, including the nutrient program, and she showed only slight improvement. Finally, we began testing her for allergies, without success, until we used a progesterone extract. The reaction was severe: crying, anxiety, and jittery nerves. With treatment, the anxiety and other problems went away completely. Progesterone-extract therapy seems to work all month long for Kim, with a dramatic calming effect.

The Allergy Quiz

When we suspect a patient has underlying allergies either as a cause or in combination with their PMS, we suggest the patient fill out our allergy questionnaire. (You will find an allergy checklist at the back of this book.) This questionnaire is designed to provide specific information on whether a person has allergies and what types of allergies may be present.

Allergies can take the form of a variety of symptoms—both physical and emotional/psychological. We have found it important to consider the possibility of allergies in patients who do not respond to the nutritional program and who have some indications that allergies exist.

We specifically use the questionnaire to help determine the nature and extent of the allergic condition of a patient. If you suspect allergy as a component of your PMS, or as a separate problem altogether, you may want to fill it out and see what patterns develop. For example, if you discover that you have specific allergy symptoms but only in the spring and fall, then chances are your allergies may be limited to pollens that are seasonal. If you discover that some types of chemicals, such as those found in cleaning products, bother you whenever you come in contact with them, then you may have a more specific, year-round allergy.

You may find that as you think about some of the questions and make observations, you will discover hidden allergies or sensitivities. Many people have no conscious awareness of the connection between food, molds and certain chemicals, and their symptoms.

In any case, if you suspect that allergies exist, we suggest you seek treatment for them. In our experience, the best type of physician to treat either allergies or *Candida albicans* infections are those trained in the field of environmental medicine. For further information about finding an environmental medicine specialist, please see the appendix.

8

WHAT CAN YOU DO UNTIL THE PROGRAM WORKS?

The nutritional approach to PMS is a process of build-up. Even if you see significant relief in the first month, you'll still have some symptoms to deal with. Following are techniques to help relieve the tension meanwhile.

FACE THE FACTS

Sometimes you are mean and moody, but there's a reason for it. You can't ignore your feelings. If you are irritable for two weeks out of the month, you can't just hope for the best and wish it away (as you probably know by now). So what can you do? While you're at the beginning of handling your PMS, sit down *during the time you are feeling good* and make a list of the kinds of symptoms that you generally get during pre-time. Do you bloat? How much? How long? How does it feel? Are you moody? What kinds of circumstances trigger a mood swing? Is there anyone or anything in particular, or any particular set of events that gets you going? Is there a particular time of day when you are at your most or least irritable? A particularly helpful or disastrous place?

If you know what is coming, if you are aware of it, expecting it, and observing it, PMS will be easier to deal with. It is vital that you become more familiar with yourself during this period of feeling good, and that you get a clear picture of what happens to you during your premenstrual time.

Take the mystery out of your pre-times, take the horror out of it. Most women are surprised—every month—when they become premenstrual. It is always bewildering, it never makes sense, it is always traumatic. It always produces guilt, and is a cause for apologies later on. Don't let that happen again. Get involved in the process of your cycle by observing what is happening and when. Chart it. Be watchful. Recognize it.

THERE IS A SOLUTION

Knowing that your premenstrual syndrome is treatable is the second step. It is useful at this time—when you are either thinking about a course of treatment or actually beginning one—to think back on how many fights or upsets you've had during PMS times, and look ahead over the next month or two. If almost every fight or traffic ticket you've gotten came three days before your period, if sleepless nights filled with self-doubt consistently come one week before your period (and the rest of the time you feel terrific), then you can understand that many of your difficulties stem from this medical problem. You may even decide that your marriage isn't quite as bad as you thought it was, or that everyday red tape is not as complicated as it had seemed.

LOOK OVER YOUR CALENDAR

Prepare yourself. Check your calendar to see what is planned over the next several months during your pre-times, and avoid potential disasters.

Some women cancel events that are stressful if they coincide with a pre-time, and reschedule them for other days of their cycle. The idea is to minimize the stresses during your premenstrual time. If possible, plan for it.

GET YOUR FAMILY TO HELP

Here you are, realizing you have PMS, wanting to try to handle it. You go to a doctor to make sure there are no underlying medical complications. What next?

The first thing you should do is sit down with your family or other close friends and explain what is going on. If possible, chart your symptoms for one month and show them this chart. You might say, "Look, I think this is what is going on with me. I never realized it before, but looking back it is clear that I've always had problems just before my period comes. So I'm going to try to work out a program that will help it."

Let your loved one(s) know when you are going into your pre-time. In fact, alert them in advance if possible. "Next Thursday is about when I usually get premenstrual. I hope I don't, but I may say things that sound worse than what I actually mean. I may be snappy, or I may fly off the handle. I may not be as patient as I mean to be." Preferably, the family will not walk on eggshells, but neither will they take things personally if you get irritable. The big difference between this month and other months may simply be that this time, you and your loved ones are more aware of what is going on.

Often, it is especially difficult for children who have to deal with their mother's premenstrual times. They tend to think, "What did *I* do to make her so mad at me?" When a child asks for help and Mom responds with frustration, perhaps with anger, maybe even fury, it is easy for the youngster to think that he or she did something wrong. The children often think there is something wrong with them. They see no rational reason why they were yelled at. Often, they try to make up for it, to make Mom feel better. This, too, is confusing and frustrating if it has little or no lasting effect. Mom feels better one minute, but then is furious again the next. The child often ends up feeling guilty, bewildered and insecure. Even adults feel that way. A husband may think, "This is not the woman I fell in love with . . ."

It is important that you sit these people down and explain the process to them, explain that PMS is a medical problem. Usually, discovering the problem and seeking treatment is a big move towards an eventual cure. Moreover, families are usually very supportive. We have had increasing numbers of husbands who call or write to us wanting information about PMS for their wives. Or they come in themselves to learn more about it, or bring their wives here. It is a tremendous boost when you can get support from someone close to you. It is also a tremendous boost for you to know that you are O.K. and will be getting even better, that you have a correctible medical problem, that you are not crazy, neurotic, or miserably unhappy because of them.

The biggest disaster is when a premenstrual mother and a premenstrual daughter are living in the same house. This explosive combination occurs frequently. It can be especially dramatic if they are premenstrual at the same time. This situation is surprisingly common as studies have shown that some women living in close proximity for more than a few months tend to synchronize their cycles and menstruate together. (We're not sure why this happens, but many women have reported it happening.)

If, on the other hand, the mother goes through her pre-time and the daughter isn't going through hers, then it seems as if the mother is a shrew and the daughter is constantly setting her off. Then the mother comes out of it and the daughter goes into her pre-time, resulting in the same pattern in the opposite direction; the daughter becomes the shrew and the mother constantly sets her off. Obviously, the relationship suffers great damage.

Does everyone get violent? Of course not. Symptoms of PMS can be inwardly tense as well as outwardly dramatic; either way they are distressing. Often, we see an adolescent who is a little quiet, a little withdrawn, maybe a little crabby. Perhaps she isn't doing as well as she could in school, or has difficulty concentrating. These kinds of symptoms are mild compared to the kinds of reactions that other people may have, yet they are major in the sense that the PMS is a slow, insidious problem for the adolescent.

Premenstrual high school students tend to get into trouble at school because of discipline problems during their PMS times. "You're hanging out with the wrong people." "You're not studying hard enough." "Where's your motivation?" "Don't you want to get into a good college?" All sorts of imaginative explanations are given by the concerned adults, but PMS is often the underlying problem—not the friends, not the school, and not the family life. Teenagers also tend to be terribly weight conscious, especially when they bloat up premenstrually, and may end up going on diets that destroy their health, when what they really need is better nutrition during these years—and especially premenstrually.

WHAT ABOUT AN UNHELPFUL FAMILY?

Getting your family to be supportive isn't always easy. What about the husband who "doesn't want to know" about PMS or your problems, who doesn't believe that PMS exists or that you have problems with it?

This phenomenon is complicated by the fact that women who have PMS often feel different and "out of it," plagued by Jekyll-and-Hyde feelings, easy prey to self-doubt. They may not trust their own judgment, particularly if their families are unsympathetic and unsupportive. Because they often say or do things they later regret, or react in a manner more pronounced than would have been appropriate, they tend to feel guilty. A woman with PMS will frequently question her own feelings if she has no outside support, and will often give up trying to get better.

What motivates a husband or other family member who is unsympathetic? Sometimes it is simply that they do not want anything to be wrong with someone they love. In the psychiatric field, we are frequently faced with this situation. "There's nothing wrong with my daughter, she just needs to work harder," is a common reaction. "There's nothing wrong with her, she just needs a good stiff drink before dinner to calm her down." "There's nothing wrong with my wife. She brings this on herself."

People commonly think that unless there is a clear-cut medical problem with a name, then there is no sickness, no disease or ill health. This is one reason why it is imperative for the health of women that PMS comes to be recognized by the population at large, so that even the most unsympathetic, closed-minded mate will accept it. As a society, we still have not fully accepted problems that entail emotional symptoms; usually, medical problems are considered valid only if there is some overt physical symptom, like a fever or stomachache. By doing this we have cut ourselves off at the neck, not permitting any other symptoms to count.

The woman with an unsympathetic husband has to get a handle on the problem herself—with or without her husband's support. PMS will not get better by itself, and once she is no longer premenstrual she can reassess the relationship to try to ascertain *why* there was no support.

People are sometimes terribly afraid of change—even a change for the better. A clearly medical problem cannot be argued with. When a physician tells a family that a woman has arthritis, it is unlikely that anyone will disbelieve it. But when the problem has emotional symptoms, or is one for which there are no medical tests, many people will deny that it exists. They often fear change because they fear loss of control.

Sometimes, in situations where the family has gotten used to the woman being "different" for several days or weeks out of every month, we see husbands who are hostile to treatment programs for their wives. The family has identified her as "the patient" and built its *modus operandi* around that role. If you take her out of the patient role, the family's routine is upset, roles get confused. It can require massive adjustments for the rest of the family. The changes may be positive ones, but even positive changes are not always welcome simply because they are changes.

SUMMARY OF GETTING STARTED

Check with your physician and get tests for a complete blood count, urinalysis, blood chemistries, and thyroid screen to be sure that there are no underlying problems. Enlist your physician as a partner in your care. Help him/her help you with the ideas we've given you.

Monitor your symptoms for at least one month, if possible, using the diary. Get a sense of what your symptoms are—and be specific. When do they occur? How bad are they? How long do they last?

Discuss PMS with your family. Talk to them about the underlying causes of PMS, the kinds of symptoms women generally have, and the kinds of symptoms that you have in particular. Talk to them about the research being done to help PMS, and the nutritional approach. If you decide to use the nutritional approach to help yourself, explain the program to your family.

Buy the vitamins and nutrients in small quantities, on a trial basis.

Organize a vitamin box for yourself. When you are taking a variety of nutrients, it can be extremely helpful to organize them. Rather than having to open ten bottles of vitamins every morning and four every evening, organize them once a week or once a month in a vitamin box, which is also simple to pack if you are going away. We recommend that women buy a vitamin box and label it for each vitamin and the dosage. This seems to simplify the matter of taking vitamins every day.If you can find an attractive looking container, it can make it even more enjoyable.

Set up an exercise program for yourself that includes some stretching and some aerobics.

Always try to take the nutrients at the same time every morning and every evening. Work it into your daily routine so you will not miss days through forgetting.

Take five minutes before going to sleep every night to fill out your diary. It doesn't take long, and is invaluable in analyzing the progress of your treatment course and in making adjustments to the nutrients.

Start slowly on low dosages and work your way up to higher dosages. Always check your diary to evaluate which symptoms have improved, which have gotten worse, and how this correlates with the dosages of nutrients you have been taking.

Talk to other women about PMS. It is fascinating and enlightening to learn about other women's experiences, how they have been helped, what they are doing now. Most women find it tremendously exciting to talk to other women who have or have had PMS and to find out first-hand that they really aren't alone. On a more formal level, workshops or support groups are a useful experience.

Because PMS symptoms often have an emotional component, it is crucial to talk to other women; it can be a huge step towards diminishing the feelings of frustration and guilt, and the sense that you are crazy. In addition, sharing methods of coping, ways of dealing with other people and experiences are, as in any other illness, a good way to begin to work things out. It's a chance to share your feelings and to express yourself, to get a load off your mind.

Talking to other women with PMS always helps. We see it all the time in our waiting room, where patients get together and start telling each other their life stories, their worst secrets. It is a source of reassurance.

Most women who have PMS have suffered with it for a long time; treatment will not be instantaneous. You will have to keep this in mind, especially if you start the nutrients just before you get your period. Commit yourself to getting rid of the PMS problem and improving your health, to living a more productive, energetic life. Commit yourself to becoming your own advocate, to becoming aware of your own body and its messages. Keep up your diaries, and chart your symptoms.

The key to success with the nutrient program is being observant. Look for a percentage of improvement. Always be aware of yourself, of *why* you are exercising, *why* you are avoiding certain foods, *why* you are taking the nutritional supplements. You are doing all of this so that your PMS problems will not continue to resurface every month. They are steps you are taking towards good health.

9

STAND UP AND
BE COUNTED

"Can I bring my husband here?" "Can you explain to my family that I'm not crazy?" "Would you be willing to call my boyfriend and explain that this is a medical problem?" Most family members who come to our workshops, or who come to us privately for more information, are extremely interested and excited about being able to help. What is more, they learn. They learn about the physiology of PMS and learn that it can be treated, which relieves their fears.

Women who have PMS, and their families, are often living in a nightmare, yet that very nightmare leaves them unable or unwilling to deal with the reasons for this monthly chaos. It is unusual for a premenstrual woman to be able to sit down with husband, friends, or children and say, honestly and self-confidently, "Look, I know that two weeks out of the month I'm a basketcase. But I think it has something to do with my period. . . . I don't know what it is, but I think we need to figure out some way to deal with it." Instead, there is a tendency to try to make up for the premenstrual time by being super good, super patient, super everything for the rest of the time. Usually, it is a failed attempt and when the next PMS time comes along, the effect is even worse.

Said one woman, "I went to my doctor so many times, asking if there wasn't some kind of blood test I could take to figure out what was wrong with me." The doctor's response was typical for those physicians who have not yet discovered the new PMS-related research. "He said that I should take mood elevators, and that I should go to a psychiatrist. Do you think I was going to tell my family that *I* was right and that the *doctor* was off base?" She did not tell her family about her PMS until after she had learned to control it because she felt they would not believe her.

Usually, after a premenstrual episode, everyone in the family willingly forgets about it. They are usually so relieved that ignoring the problem is reflexive. They relax, they go through their normal life patterns. Then the problems start again. Often, the end of a premenstrual time sees the woman trying to make up with everyone in her family, apologizing for "going to extremes" (again), and promising (again) to try harder. Often, she will hear "Why can't you always be like this?" or "I just don't understand you. Sometimes you are so reasonable—and at other times, you're just a different person."

But when her next pre-time comes, and she is again moody, irritable, and "unreasonable," she has broken her promises. That makes it even worse. "Here we go again," "Get off my back," and "Give me a break," are commonly heard.

When the premenstrual time is over, everyone wants to forget about it. No one likes the idea that Mom was crazy for two weeks. No one wants to face it, no one wants to remember or accept it. If they ignore it, it will go away. They ignore it, and it does go away—for two weeks, maybe three, and then it comes back.

Some people build an entire relationship around this kind of premenstrual cycle. They fight for a week or two and then they spend the next two or three weeks recovering and making up. Then they fight again.

It is a never-ending cycle while the premenstrual syndrome exists, and it tends to build up in intensity. Many relationships cannot tolerate it. Often the woman feels intense guilt because she is being accused of things that are true; the man is often terribly confused. Sometimes abuse becomes a component in the relationship. Said one husband, "I do not want to hit her because I don't believe in violence. But sometimes Sheila is so deliberately provocative that, I'm ashamed to say, I do hit her. It starts with an argument, and she usually throws something. . . . I'd like to say it was just self-defense, but the truth is that I'm also so angry myself, by this time, that I have no control." (Lever, J., *Premenstrual Tension*, New York: McGraw Hill, 1982).

Why is it so hard for people to pin PMS down, to realize that this is a set of symptoms that come, like clockwork, every month? Why does it take women, and then their families, years before they make the connections?

Let's contrast PMS with a medical symptom like a sore throat. What happens when you have a sore throat? First, it occurs as a defined physical problem. "The problem is here, in my throat. It began at 3'oclock. It hurts here, especially when I swallow." The doctor looks down your throat, takes a throat culture, and sends the culture to a lab for testing. He writes out a prescription for antibiotics if the lab results indicate strep infection. A sore throat has a name and a form and a physicality; it usually has a remedy, or a series of remedial procedures.

The entire process goes like this: 1) you feel pain; 2) you contact the doctor or other expert; 3) the doctor listens to your problem, examines you, and corroborates your analysis.

But PMS symptoms are evident in the emotional framework as often or even more often than they are in the physical framework. They do not have a clear beginning, middle or end. Although there are biological bases, the symptoms do not seem scientifically real because they cannot be measured, they cannot be prodded and tested, and they can be difficult to separate from specific circumstances. The medical world has only just started to map psychological symptoms, which are so much harder to pinpoint than the more obvious or gross physical symptoms. A rash is far easier to discern than the subtle destruction of a person's sense of self-worth, although both can be the result of physical problems.

Also, the subject of menstruation itself is still not entirely acceptable. It is no longer taboo as it was thirty years ago. But daughters still avoid telling their fathers, for instance, when they get their period, and confide in their girlfriends in hushed whispers in the school hallways. Women today may be more liberated than their forebears, but the message that menstruation should be kept secret still lingers.

This lesson of privacy, combined with the subtle nature of emotional symptoms and changes, hinders many women from making the obvious connections between their emotional and/or physical state and their menstrual cycle. Instead, they tend to think that they're emotionally disturbed and that there's something inherently wrong with them.

In addition, there are often background circumstances that make irritability and other symptoms seem reasonable, rather than unreasonable, and so cloud the issue. Take the case of Barbara and Joe. Barbara was given progesterone as a treatment for prolonged spotting. Within days, she became premenstrual, although she had never had PMS problems before.

"She was impossible," recalls Joe. "She was two people, not the person I married. She was awful. She was also right. I mean, she'd get all bent out of shape over some dumb thing that I'd done, or neglected to do, and the thing was, she was right. What could I say? Like, I'd use her car and forget to put gas in it and she'd have to make a separate trip out for gas. But she would get so mad, it was out of all proportion to the incident. How mad can you get about a trip to the gas station? On the other hand, it takes a good half an hour to go and come back, so she was right, too."

Joe and the children convinced Barbara to stop the treatments and return to her "normal" self, which she did, deciding that anything was better than PMS, especially since Joe was likely to make more mistakes in the future, and the children were imperfect sometimes, too.

REACTIONS TO PMS

Premenstrual syndrome has been sucessfully used as a defense in the British courts to reduce charges or sentencing for women arrested for violent crimes. In one case, for instance, a woman ran her car into her lover and killed him, but was allowed to plead guilty to manslaughter, rather than murder, on the grounds of "diminished responsibility" due to PMS. While some applaud the ethic of pleading diminished responsibility or capacity, or temporary insanity, due to PMS, others see it as a giant step backwards in the struggle for women's rights.

Whether PMS should be used as a legal defense—and whether "temporary insanity" itself should be used as a legal defense—is a complicated moral issue. Yet the use of PMS as a legal defense, and thus its admission that premenstrual women are temporarily insane or of diminished responsibility has become central to the feminist acceptance (or non-acceptance) of PMS as a real problem for half of womankind. Surprisingly, some feminists look at premenstrual syndrome as something to deny, as something that threatens women's right to be treated as mens' equals, with equal rights, capabilities and responsibilities.

The problem that some feminists are having with PMS is that they accept the definition of premenstrual syndrome as a "woman's problem" instead of as a "medical problem."

Recently, there was a TV talk show in which a feminist group, one that was antagonistic to the publicity surrounding premenstrual syndrome and the bad name it gave women, was pitted against a very conservative doctor who was known to make statements to the effect that "all women should stay home and not take jobs away from men," and that "women should accept their God-given role as mothers and wives and not try to do things they are 'unable' to do, like work in construction, in corporate business, or as athletes." One of the feminist women denied PMS as a medical issue, saying that it is a gender problem, something that is natural to women—and therefore should not be "fussed" over. She felt that the publicity surrounding PMS is setting the stage for a new round of gender discrimination. She was angry that the courts had upheld PMS as a legal defense and was concerned that one of the subtle results would be that women in general might be seen as unreliable, subject to fits of violence, and/or periods of lowered capacity. (All the statistics show that premenstrual women with PMS are considerably less violent than men are all the time.) The doctor, in his paternalistic way, was endorsing precisely the view that the feminists were most wary of: That women are "weaker, more emotional, less competent than men, as evidenced by premenstrual syndrome, and that they need the protection of men for those times when they are hysterical."

We feel that the real situation is very much different from this scenario. As long as PMS is considered to be a gender issue and not a medical one, we are at its mercy. As a medical issue, PMS can be overcome.

Let us explain. If it is a gender issue, something *natural* and *acceptable* to women, then half of the women in our society will never be able to feel as good as they should, half of them will not be able to demand equal pay for equal responsibility, will never be able to stop struggling with themselves during the days when they are fatigued, lethargic, depressed, or working with "diminished capacity." If we accept PMS as a gender issue, we are accepting the logic of those who shrug and say, "Why should I hire a woman when I can hire a man?"

If we refuse to accept that PMS actually exists, we are denying women with premenstrual syndrome the right to good health.

PMS is a correctible medical problem. Yes, it is common. Between 80 and 90 percent of the women who have come to us with PMS have been treated successfully. Once it is corrected, there is no such thing as diminished capacity or diminished responsibility. These are highly competent—and self-assured—women.

You wouldn't say to a male with heart disease, "That's just part of being a man. Better get used to it." No. You work to help them and immediately begin therapy because you want the person to get better.

Why, then, do we say to women with PMS, "That's just the way you are. It's part of being a woman."? Why do we say "You are just spoiled and you want people to feel sorry for you."? Likewise, we do not say to a male with heart disease, "You don't really have a heart problem. You're just looking for sympathy."

Statistics revealing the number of work days lost by women who suffer from PMS, how much PMS costs the economy, or how much it costs a company, are all used to keep women either out of the workforce altogether or working at low wages. The statistics are valid; it is true that women with PMS lose more work time, do not make as accurate judgments, are not as reliable as they would be if they did not have PMS. The point is, that the condition is a medically correctible imbalance. It is inexcusable for our society to try to keep women from getting help. To get rid of a medical problem that has been used to keep women down is a goal that, if reached, would be of enormous benefit not only to the women involved, but to all of society.

The women we know who have corrected their PMS problems are more productive, stronger, more self-confident women now than they ever were before. They are women who can rightfully demand equal pay for work of equal value—and they do. They are women who can stand up and be counted, all month long.

APPENDIX

BIBLIOGRAPHY
for
THE BIOCHEMISTRY OF PMS

Atton-Chamla, A., G. Faure, and J.-R. Goudard. "Premenstrual Syndrome and Atopy." *Pharmatherapeutica,* 2 (1980), 481-86.

Abraham, G.E., and M.M. Lubran. "Serum and Red Cell Magnesium Levels in Patients with Premenstrual Tension." *Am. J. Clin. Nutr.,* 34 (1981), 2364-366.

Abraham, G.E., U.L.F.D. Schwartz, and M.M. Lubran. "Effect of Vitamin B_6 on Plasma and Red Blood Cell Magnesium Levels in Premenstrual Women." *Ann. Clin. Lab. Sci.,* 11 (1981), 333-36.

Brush, M.G. "Efamol (Evening Primrose Oil) in the Treatment of Premenstrual Syndrome." *The Clinical Uses of Essential Fatty Acids."* Ed. D.F. Horobin, Eden Press, Montreal, 1982.

Brush, M.G., S.J. Watson, D.F. Horrobin, and M.S. Manku. "Abnormal Essential Fatty Acid Levels in Plasma of Women with Premenstrual Syndrom." *Amer. J. Obstet. Gynec.,* in press, 1984.

Horrobin, D.F. "The Role of Essential Fatty Acids and Prostaglandins in the Premenstrual Syndrome." *J. Reprod. Med.,* 28 (1983), 465-68.

Horrobin, D.F., M.G. Brush, K. Callender, P.E. Preece and R.E. Mansel. "Abnormalities in Plasma Essential Fatty Acid Levels in Women with Premenstrual syndrome and with Non-malignant Breast Disease." Submitted for publication, 1984.

Ockerman, P.-A., and I. Bachrack. "Essential Fatty Acids in the Treatment of the Premenstrual Syndrome." Submitted for publication, 1984.

Preece, P.E., J.I. Hanslip, L. Gilbert, D. Walker, N.L. Pashby, R.E. Mansel, B. Evans and L.E. Hughes. "Evening Primrose Oil (Efamol) for Mastalgia." *Clinical Uses of Essential Fatty Acids.* Ed. D.F. Horrobin, Eden Press, Montreal, 1982.

Sampson, G.A. "Premenstrual Syndrome: A Double Blind Controlled Trial of Progesterone and Placebo." *Br. J. Psychiatry,* 130 (1979), 265-74.

Wright, S. and J.L. Burton. "Oral Evening Primrose Oil Improves Atopic Eczema." *Lancet,* 2 (1982), 1120-122.

Ylikorkala, O., J. Puolakka, L. Makarainen and L. Viinikka. "6-keto-prostaglandin F1-alpha and thromboxane B_1 in Premenstrual Syndrome: The Effect of Treatment with Prostaglandin Synthesis Precursors." Submitted for publication, 1984.

REFERENCES

Allen, P. and D. Fortino. *Cycles: Every Woman's Guide to Menstruation.* Pinnacle Books, 1983.

Brody, J. *Jane Brody's Nutrition Book.* Bantam Books, 1982.

Buddoff, Penny Wise. *No More Menstrual Cramps and Other Good News.* Penguin Books, 1981.

Dalton, K. *The Premenstrual Syndrome and Progesterone Therapy.* Year Book Medical Publishers, Inc., 1977.

Gershon, Mark. *A Choice of Heroes.*

Health Quest's Nutrition and Lifestyle Handbook. Health Quest Inc., 1982.

Lever, J. *Premenstrual Tension.* New York: McGraw Hill, 1982.

Mozalla, Caroline. *The Premenstrual Syndrome.*

Pfeiffer, Carol. *Mental and Elemental Nutrients.* 1975.

Physician's Desk Reference.

Shreeve, Caroline. *The Premenstrual Syndrome.* Thorsons, 1983.

Truss, Orian. C. *The Missing Diagnosis.* O.C. Truss, Birmingham, Alabama, 1983.

NOTES

1. A. Labrun and K. Rothman, unpublished study, Rochester, N.Y., 1982. With permission.
2. R.A. McCance, M.C. Luff and E.E. Widdowson, "Irritability During the Menstrual Cycle," *J. Hyg.,* 37 (1938), 571-611. With permission.
3. *Proceedings of the Royal Society of Medicine,* 59 (1966), 1014-16. With permission.
4. Ibid.
5. C.M. Tonks, P.H. Rack and M.D. Rose, "Attempted Suicide and the Menstrual Cycle," *J. Psych. Res.,* 2, 4 (1968), 319-23. With permission.
6. Institute of Food Technologies, "Scientific Status summary on Caffeine." First printed in the *Valley Advocate,* 17 August 1983. With permission.
7. Ann M. Holmes, *Nutrition and Vitamins,* Facts on File, Inc., 1983. With permission.
8. *Consumer Reports,* "Salt and High Blood Pressure," 44 (1979), 147-49. With permission.

OTHER BOOKS ON PMS

Budoff. *No More Menstrual Cramps and Other Good News.* Penguin Books, 1982.

Dalton, K. *PMS and Progesterone Therapy,* 2nd Edition. Yearbook of Medicine, 1984.

Dalton, K. *Once a Month,* Hunter House, 1979.

Harrison, M. *Self-Help for PMS,* Matrix Press, 1982.

Norris, R.V. and C. Sullivan. *PMS: The Cause and Cure of the Syndrome that Affects 500 Million Women,* Rawson Assoc., 1983.

Rappoport, W. *PMS: A Self-Help Guide,* Compact Books, 1984.

Schreeve, C. *PMS: The Curse That Can Be Cured,* Thorsons Ltd., 1983.

Wade, C. *Carlson Wade's PMS Book,* Keats Press, 1984.

United States and Canada
The following organizations may be of some assistance to you.

The American Academy of Environmental Medicine
P.O. Box 16106
Denver, Colorado
U.S.A.   80216

Premenstrual Syndrome Centre
1077 N. Service Road
Applewood Plaza
Mississauga, Ontario   L4Y 1A6
Tel: (416) 273-7770

National Institute of Nutrition
P.O. Box 879
Stittsville, Ontario   K0A 3G0
Tel: (613) 836-1287

In the U.K.
If you are seeking advice on PMT, you should initially contact your general practitioner, who can refer you to a PMT clinic operating at your nearest hospital or Well-Woman Centre. Other useful addresses and telephone numbers are:

PMT Advisory Service
Box Number 268
Hove, Sussex   BN2 1RW
Tel: Brighton 771366

Women's Health Information Centre
55, Featherstone Street
London EC1
Tel: 01-251 6580

Women's Health Concern
16, Seymour Street
London W1
Tel: 01-602 6669

The Family Planning Association
27, Mortimer Street
London W1
Tel: 01-636 7866

AN ALLERGY CHECKLIST

Check those symptoms that apply to you

- [ ] itchy eyes
- [ ] light sensitivity
- [ ] eye infections
- [ ] ear infections
- [ ] ear drainage
- [ ] blocked ear
- [ ] earaches
- [ ] sinus infections
- [ ] frequent sore throat
- [ ] cough
- [ ] wheezing
- [ ] frequent colds
- [ ] shortness of breath
- [ ] chest pain
- [ ] rapid heart beat
- [ ] constipation
- [ ] diarrhea
- [ ] excessive gas
- [ ] bloating
- [ ] nausea
- [ ] stomachaches
- [ ] rectal itching
- [ ] eczema
- [ ] itching
- [ ] redness
- [ ] shingles
- [ ] rash
- [ ] insomnia
- [ ] headaches
- [ ] seizures
- [ ] anxiety
- [ ] professional psychiatric help
- [ ] depression
- [ ] regular

- [ ] post-nasal drip
- [ ] stuffed-up nose
- [ ] bloody nose
- [ ] cankers
- [ ] chapped lips
- [ ] fever blisters
- [ ] throat plate itches
- [ ] hoarseness
- [ ] deviated septum
- [ ] heart attack
- [ ] heart murmur
- [ ] bronchitis
- [ ] pneumonia
- [ ] emphysema
- [ ] high blood pressure
- [ ] use of laxatives
- [ ] use of antacids
- [ ] heartburn
- [ ] colitis
- [ ] vomiting
- [ ] ulcer
- [ ] irregular heart beats
- [ ] dry skin
- [ ] boils
- [ ] sores
- [ ] hives
- [ ] contact dermatitis
- [ ] seborrheic dermatitis
- [ ] crying spells
- [ ] excessive appetite
- [ ] low appetite
- [ ] hospitalized for psychiatric illness
- [ ] suicidal feelings
- [ ] low energy

- [ ] problems associated with birth control use
- [ ] pre-period cramps
- [ ] pre-period mood changes
- [ ] pre-period bloating
- [ ] fluid retention
- [ ] kidney infections
- [ ] trichomonas
- [ ] acne
- [ ] excessive bleeding during period
- [ ] period cramps
- [ ] pre-period headaches
- [ ] breasts tender pre-period
- [ ] pain with intercourse
- [ ] yeast infections
- [ ] herpes
- [ ] frigidity

PRE-MENSTRUAL SYNDROME – WEEKLY DIARY

Start Date: _____   Finish Date: _____

Day of Cycle .... Day___	Day___	Day___	Day___	Day___	Day___	Day___
Nutrients:	am | pm	am | pm	am | pm	am | pm	am | pm	am | pm	am | pm

Day of the Week .... ( )   ( )   ( )   ( )   ( )   ( )   ( )

Indicate Symptom Intensity
(1–10) 1 = Best; 10 = Worst

	am | pm	am | pm	am | pm	am | pm	am | pm	am | pm	am | pm
Acne							
Anxiety							
Bloating							
Breast Tenderness							
Constipation; Diarrhea							
Cramps							
Crying (No. of times)							
Depression							
Energy Level							
Headache							
Irritability; Mood Changes							
Sexual Responsiveness							
Lower Back Pain							
Nausea; Vomiting							
Vaginal Discharge							

Alcohol (# of oz.)							
Appetite (1–10)							
Cravings (1–10)							
Exercise (# of min.)							
The Pill (✔)							
Sleep (# of hours)							
Temperature							
Weight							
Days of Menstruation (✔)							

PATIENT'S NAME _____

PRE-MENSTRUAL SYNDROME – WEEKLY DIARY

Start Date: _____   Finish Date: _____

Day of Cycle	Day___		Day___		Day___		Day___		Day___		Day___		Day___	
Nutrients:	am	pm	am	pm	am	pm	am	pm	am	pm	am	pm	am	pm
_____														
Day of the Week	( )		( )		( )		( )		( )		( )		( )	

Indicate Symptom Intensity
(1–10) 1 = Best; 10 = Worst

	am	pm	am	pm	am	pm	am	pm	am	pm	am	pm	am	pm
Acne														
Anxiety														
Bloating														
Breast Tenderness														
Constipation; Diarrhea														
Cramps														
Crying (No. of times)														
Depression														
Energy Level														
Headache														
Irritability; Mood Changes														
Sexual Responsiveness														
Lower Back Pain														
Nausea; Vomiting														
Vaginal Discharge														

Alcohol (# of oz.)														
Appetite (1–10)														
Cravings (1–10)														
Exercise (# of min.)														
The Pill (✔)														
Sleep (# of hours)														
Temperature														
Weight														
Days of Menstruation (✔)														

PATIENT'S NAME _____

PRE-MENSTRUAL SYNDROME – WEEKLY DIARY

Start Date: _____   Finish Date: _____

Day of Cycle ·········· Day___	Day___		Day___		Day___		Day___		Day___		Day___		Day___	
Nutrients:	am	pm	am	pm	am	pm	am	pm	am	pm	am	pm	am	pm
_____														
_____														
_____														
_____														
_____														
_____														
_____														
_____														
Day of the Week ········	(	)	(	)	(	)	(	)	(	)	(	)	(	)

Indicate Symptom Intensity
(1–10) 1 = Best; 10 = Worst

	am	pm	am	pm	am	pm	am	pm	am	pm	am	pm	am	pm
Acne														
Anxiety														
Bloating														
Breast Tenderness														
Constipation; Diarrhea														
Cramps														
Crying (No. of times)														
Depression														
Energy Level														
Headache														
Irritability; Mood Changes														
Sexual Responsiveness														
Lower Back Pain														
Nausea; Vomiting														
Vaginal Discharge														
Alcohol (# of oz.)														
Appetite (1–10)														
Cravings (1–10)														
Exercise (# of min.)														
The Pill (✔)														
Sleep (# of hours)														
Temperature														
Weight														
Days of Menstruation (✔)														

PATIENT'S NAME _____

PRE-MENSTRUAL SYNDROME – WEEKLY DIARY

Start Date: _____   Finish Date: _____

Day of Cycle	Day___		Day___		Day___		Day___		Day___		Day___		Day___	
Nutrients:	am	pm	am	pm	am	pm	am	pm	am	pm	am	pm	am	pm

Day of the Week .... ( )   ( )   ( )   ( )   ( )   ( )   ( )

Indicate Symptom Intensity
(1–10) 1 = Best; 10 = Worst

	am	pm	am	pm	am	pm	am	pm	am	pm	am	pm	am	pm
Acne														
Anxiety														
Bloating														
Breast Tenderness														
Constipation; Diarrhea														
Cramps														
Crying (No. of times)														
Depression														
Energy Level														
Headache														
Irritability; Mood Changes														
Sexual Responsiveness														
Lower Back Pain														
Nausea; Vomiting														
Vaginal Discharge														

Alcohol (# of oz.)														
Appetite (1–10)														
Cravings (1–10)														
Exercise (# of min.)														
The Pill (✔)														
Sleep (# of hours)														
Temperature														
Weight														
Days of Menstruation (✔)														

PATIENT'S NAME _____

Printed in Canada